"The Physician's Hand"

"The Physician's Hand"

Work Culture and Conflict in American Nursing

Barbara Melosh

Temple University Press
Philadelphia

To my parents:
Gurlie J. Melosh, R.N.
and
William D. Melosh, M.D.

Temple University Press, Philadelphia 19122
© 1982 by Temple University
Published 1982
Printed in the United States of America

Library of Congress Cataloging in Publication Data

Melosh, Barbara.
  The physician's hand.

  Includes bibliographical references and index.
  1. Nursing—United States—History. I. Title.
[DNLM: 1. History of nursing. WY 11.1 M528p]
RT4.M44 1982   610.73′0973   82-10537
ISBN 0-87722-278-9 cloth, 0-87722-290-8 paper

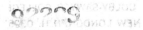

CONTENTS

ACKNOWLEDGMENTS

I am happy to acknowledge the many people who have helped me to think and write about nurses and nursing.

My mother is a nurse and my father is a doctor. Their enthusiasm for nursing and medicine was the source of my own early interest, and influenced my decision to write on nursing.

The research for this study took place in a number of libraries. In each, my work was smoothed by pleasant and efficient staff members. The Nursing Archives and general collection at Boston University's Mugar Library provided most of the materials for this study. I have a special fondness for the Providence Public Library, where the long-suffering staff patiently transported volumes of nursing journals from remote corners of the stacks. The Schlesinger Library at Radcliffe and the Boston and New York Public Libraries each contained memoirs and novels unavailable elsewhere. The Library of Congress—the mother of us all—yielded new sources and provided office space as I revised the manuscript.

Three grants gave me time at different stages of the project. The Ellen H. Richards fellowship of the American Association of University Women helped me to launch the dissertation on which this book is based. The University of Wisconsin Summer Fund supported the first months of my revisions. The Smithsonian Institution's post-doctoral fellowship supported a precious year off, and at the National Museum of American History, I benefited from the insights and company of a new set of colleagues.

Elaine Haste and Susie Cox expertly typed the final copy, and cheerfully shared the many technical details of arranging the manuscript in finished form.

At Brown University, Mari Jo Buhle, my advisor, provided support, encouragement, close readings, and stimulating criticism at every stage. Judith N. Lasker brought the perspective of medical sociology to her own careful readings and helpful criticism. A. Hunter Dupree was open to a kind of argument that strays far from traditional history of science, and offered insightful comments and suggestions.

Many nurses have contributed to this study. In Providence, Rhode Island, I worked at the dialysis unit of a large teaching hospital, an experience that led me to study the history of nursing. My own initiation and experience in hospital work alerted me to the complex mechanisms of work culture, and taught me its critical role in getting the work done. The nurses there answered my endless questions, taught me how to manage the stresses of hospital work, and gave me a strong appreciation for the skills and satisfactions of nursing. They will not approve of my title: I only hope that the book itself conveys the several meanings I have seen in this much-resented phrase.

In collecting the oral histories of other nurses, I was deeply grateful to those women who shared their stories. My mother, Gurlie J. Melosh, helped me to arrange several other interviews in addition to recording her own nursing experiences.

Many colleagues have offered comments and criticism on one or more chapters. I thank Patricia Cooper, Audrey Davis, J. Rogers Hollingsworth, Judith Walzer Leavitt, Thomas J. McCormick, Sonya Michel, Ronald L. Numbers, and Deborah Warner.

Three women, close friends and historians themselves, have shaped this book and sustained me through its many stages. Christina Simmons and Judith E. Smith shared the initiation rites of graduate school with me, and our work group, formed in 1973, has seen me through nearly a decade. They have heard and read many versions of the book; their criticism and support have been, and are, essential. Susan Porter Benson has read this book in all its various manifestations; no one has been closer to the project. Her work on saleswomen and her wide knowledge of women's history and labor history have stimulated me to rethink many parts of my own work. At a difficult stage of writing, she pulled me through with steady encouragement and a wonderful sense of humor.

Finally, Gary Kulik has seen me and this project through many transformations. Our jobs have sometimes put half a continent between us: absorbed with his own writing and his work at the Smithsonian's National Museum of American History, he has not done my housework, typed the manuscript, or been at hand to cheer every paragraph. Instead, he lent his keen historical sensitivity to many discussions of nurses and nursing, and offered insightful comments on several chapters. He moved me and *"The Physician's Hand"* across the country three times, and lived with me in its final year. Together we have struggled with the complex task of joining work and love, and have shared the difficulties and rewards of both.

"The Physician's Hand"

Introduction

Women's dominance in nursing nearly equals our monopoly on motherhood: nursing has always been a woman's job. In the mid-nineteenth century, most nursing care was done at home as part of women's domestic duties. Florence Nightingale's 1860 manual, *Notes on Nursing*, was addressed to women in families and opened with the assertion, "Every woman is a nurse."[1] As medical care became more complex and more tied to hospitals, nursing gradually separated from the sphere of women's domestic work and became established as paid work that required special training. Arguments of women's special fitness for nursing connected traditional domestic roles to female participation in this new category of paid labor. As one doctor wrote in 1925, "A hospital is a home for the sick, and there can be no home unless there is a woman at the head of it."[2] While these sentimental images of nursing as womanly service lingered, the actual content and practice of nursing grew increasingly specialized. In the esoteric technological setting of modern hospitals, no one would proclaim that "every woman is a nurse." But the cultural ideology of woman's place still informs medical division of labor: nearly every nurse is a woman.

Unlike most women's jobs, nursing has been characterized by the presence of an articulate and self-conscious elite. Identified with Nightingale's English hospital reforms, these leaders sought to move American nursing in the same direction. Beginning in 1873, they opened hospital schools and argued that nursing was a special skill that required such training. They struggled to establish nursing as respectable

work for middle-class women, recruiting among them to
replace the socially marginal women who had traditionally
done most of the hospital's work. They formed associations to
share their problems and to promote the cause of the "trained
nurse" to a wider audience. They sought the public legitimacy
of legal licensure to affirm and defend the nurse's skills. In
their efforts to establish educational credentials, licensure, and
employment standards, they worked to assert the control over
training and practice that is the mark of established professions.

These leaders have shaped our views and understanding
of nursing history. Highly visible and vocal, they promoted a
certain ideal of the "professional" nurse in journals, surveys,
reports, manuals, even in novels. Leaders also left a number of
histories, interpreting the development of their occupation in
the image of their own hopes and aspirations. Like their
medical colleagues, these nurses celebrated a history of progress, from "the twilight and the darkness" before Nightingale
to the triumphs of modern nursing. The heroes in these narratives are nurses' leaders, shown as dedicated reformers; the
aim and end of reform is professionalization.[3]

But sifting back through nurses' written literature and
listening to oral memoirs, we hear voices that trace the shad-
owy outlines of another history of nursing. This evidence
reveals that leaders faced considerable opposition in their own
ranks: the ideals and goals they set forth were hotly contested
by nurses themselves. Such conflict emerged as a consistent
and pervasive theme in nursing history. Bitter struggles
accompanied each proposal for new educational standards and
licensure, indicating deep divisions among nurses. In letters to
the editors of the *American Journal of Nursing*, many nurses
protested leaders' strategies and criticized their professional
ideology. Two other journals spoke for those nurses who
disagreed with their official organs. *Trained Nurse and Hospital
Review*, first published in 1888, often took a critical stance
toward the professional associations, and attracted dissenting
nurses as authors, readers, and letter-writers. The first issue of

RN: A Journal for Nurses, published in 1937, promised to follow "the expressed will of the rank and file of nurses," and noted (in 1938), "Because *RN* is independent, it is able to serve its readers freely and without prejudice. There are no ax-grinding groups to dictate its editorial policy."[4] Oral and written memoirs offer further evidence of nurses' mixed feelings about their professional leaders. Finally, in mute testimony to their alienation from official leaders, nurses stayed away from their professional associations in droves.

Resistance to professionalization was one expression of an occupational culture that developed quite outside the professional associations. Most nurses interpreted their work from a different and sometimes sharply divergent perspective. Leaders looked outward, beyond the work experience to its social context and implications. Aspiring professionals, they oriented themselves to nursing's place in the larger structure of work and sought to improve nurses' positions within the medical division of labor. Nurses on the job were sometimes threatened by the strategies leaders adopted, for the rising standards of professionalization often meant downgrading or even eliminating current practitioners. More often they were simply distant from leaders, absorbed in the exigencies and rewards of daily work. It was this shared experience, not the hope of professionalization, that shaped ordinary nurses' aspirations and ideology.

Sociologists and historians of work have noted the distinctive language, lore, and social rules that workers create on the job, and have used terms like work culture, shopfloor culture, and occupational culture to suggest the coherence and structure of these activities. Generated partly in response to specific working conditions, work culture includes adaptations or resistance to constraints imposed by managers, employers, or the work itself. Constructed from workers' accumulated experiences and their understandings of the workplace, occupational culture guides and interprets the tasks and social relations of work. The content and complex workings of occupational culture are an inextricable part of the work process itself. Common understandings and work lore mediate between the formal rules and the more ambiguous circumstances of everyday work. Occupational culture is not just an elaboration on work; it is the critical link between a job's official protocol and its actual performance. Without it, most work simply could not be done. Located at this vital juncture, occupational culture at once reveals workers' central contributions to production and suggests a powerful wedge for claiming and extending workers' control on the job. Further, it provides a structure and an ideology for such claims. More than simply reactive or narrowly functional, occupational culture also embodies workers' own definition of a good day's work, their own measures of satisfying and competent performance.[5]

Shaped in the powerful common experience of nurses' distinctive training, nursing's occupational culture was sustained, revised, reinterpreted, and passed on through networks that formed after graduation. It provided a rich source of lore, anecdotes, and prescriptions for managing the nurse's intricate relationships with patients, doctors, supervisors, and hospital administrators. Sometimes it was written down: nursing journals contain some examples, and nurses' memoirs and didactic novels offered instructive models. More often it was an oral tradition, transmitted as nurses met in registries, participated in alumnae associations or other professional groups, worked together in public health agencies or on hospital wards, and lived together in hospital nursing residences. Rooted in the apprenticeship tradition of the hospital schools, nurses' work culture valued careful craft methods, practical experience, and self-control. This was nursing's mainstream; professional ideology was an influential but minority position, even an aberration.

"The Physician's Hand" recasts nursing history from the viewpoint of nurses on the job, and places it in the context of women's history, labor history, and medical history and sociology. The title evokes three central aspects of that experience. It calls attention, first, to the relationship that defines nurses' position in the medical hierarchy. By law and custom, nurses are subordinate to physicians. At the same time, it captures the nurse's critical role in executing the physician's work. Second in the line of command, nurses are closely associated with the power and prestige of medicine. In the intricate hospital hierarchy, they reign over practical nurses and aides, orderlies, and a plethora of other auxiliary workers. Second, interpreted in a rather different way, "the physician's hand" suggests the strength and character of nurses' occupational culture, a tradition of pride in manual skills, of direct involvement with the sick, of respect for experience and often a concomitant mistrust for theory. Finally, "the physician's hand" is a phrase that symbolizes years of struggle, for nurses have never been content to define their work solely in relation to doctors. Both in professional associations and on the job, nurses have sought to claim and defend their own sphere of legitimate authority. Leaders called it professional autonomy; nurses on the job might well have named it workers' control.

Removed from the limited framework of professionalization, nursing history can provide a fresh perspective on broader issues in social history. First, nursing offers an illuminating example of the ways in which gender informs work, and conversely, how work both reproduces and transforms existing relationships of power and inequality. Medical division of labor replicates a larger sexual division of labor. At work, nurses care for helpless patients and defer to doctors just as in families women care for children and defer to fathers or husbands. But over the twentieth century, the content and cultural meaning of nursing have altered with the development of medical science and practice, with the growth of health service industries, and with women's changing prospects and life choices, especially their increasing participation in the public world of paid labor. In this history we see the complexity and diversity of sex-segregation itself; its persistence as a structure but also its shifting implications under changing conditions.[6]

Second, nurses' historical experience can add a new

dimension to our understanding of work. In the last decade, reformulations of labor history have focused on the disruption of traditional craft methods and work rhythms as the factory system superseded home production. David Montgomery, Herbert Gutman, and others have evoked the world of pre-industrial work and traced its transformation under industrial capitalism. Turning to work in the twentieth century, Daniel Nelson, Harry Braverman, and Montgomery have explored the inroads of scientific management in the workplace and the impact of rationalization on skill. While some have empha-sized the unevenness of the applications of scientific manage-ment and examined workers' resistance to it, all have por-trayed the general tendency of rationalization to dilute skill and to undermine workers' control.[7]

This important interpretation has rested on a narrow base. With few exceptions, labor historians have been preoc-cupied with artisans or skilled workers—weavers, shoemak-ers, machinists—with some forays into the experiences of workers in heavy industries—miners and steelworkers. Few have considered the implications of rationalization for women workers, despite the steadily growing number of women in the workforce. Nor have labor historians explored what may well be the central issue of the twentieth century, the develop-ment of the service industries that now dominate the economy and the labor market.[8]

More than a story of professionalization, nursing history is the story of women workers' experience in a rationalizing service industry. The reorganization of nursing care roughly paralleled the reorganization of other forms of production. It was provided first by family members for one another; then incorporated into a market economy as women began to nurse for hire in their patients' homes; then concentrated in central plants where workers were subject to close supervision and new forms of control. Hospital administrators responded to industrial plans for reorganization, seeking to standardize their plants and to rationalize the work that went on in them.

The efficiency expert and the stopwatch came to hospitals as they had come to factories, stores, and offices.

At the same time, the special conditions of medical care and of service work modified the uses and meaning of rationalization for nursing. Like other workers, nurses faced a fundamental reorganization of work that changed the content and experience of nursing. But unlike many others, they did not suffer a dilution of skill. Indeed, the changing scientific base and technological innovations of medicine gave nurses new skills and authority on the job. Rationalization also changed the social relations of work in ways that gave nurses more control. Such relations were the core of service work: the "point of production" lay in the many activities encompassed by the charge to "obey the doctor" and "do what is best for the patient." The reorganization of nursing created new possibilities for managing and interpreting nurses' traditional relationships to doctors and patients.

Nursing history suggests that social relations are themselves an integral part of the definition and defense of skill. *"The Physician's Hand"* explores the shifting configurations of those relationships and their implications for nurses' work. In private duty, the nurse worked with one patient who was also her employer, and shared the case with the doctor, who supervised her. In public health, nurses worked in agencies; patients were clients with less personal authority over the nurse, and physicians were largely absent. In hospitals, nurses entered a bureaucratic workplace. Hired by administrators and in managerial positions themselves, they directed the nursing hierarchy, established new relationships with doctors, and grew more distant from patients. Nurses' increasing technical skills were just one aspect of the complex social changes that extended their control at work.

Third, nurses' location in a larger division of labor makes their history a useful standpoint for analyzing the possibilities and limitations of women's work. Nursing is a good job for a woman: that truism reveals much about sex-segregated work.

Nursing is one of the more desirable women's jobs. It requires post-high school training and offers a modicum of economic security, both notches on the measuring stick of occupational status. Although nurses do not have the elite social backgrounds common in male professions like medicine or law, they do represent an elite among working women. Nurses have been consistently drawn from the respectable reaches of middle-class and working-class families. Their fathers are slightly more likely than fathers of other women to be professionals or managers. Nurses have been disproportionately white, either native-born or of English, Irish, Scottish, or Canadian origins. For immigrant daughters and black women, nursing has often represented and sometimes fulfilled hopes of upward mobility. But on the larger scale of the whole workforce, nurses drop to a somewhat lower position. They have borne the same burdens as workers in other "women's" jobs: low salaries, obligatory deference to male superiors, an association with menial or "dirty" work. Thus, although nurses do not represent a cross-section of working women, their occupation still provides a rich example of the experience and meaning of women's work.

Finally, nurses' history alerts us to the complexities of working women's consciousness. It counters the common notion of women's passivity in the workplace. Whether seen through the self-conscious narratives of nursing history or through the social historian's evidence of nurses' activities on the job, nurses' historical experience reveals women's vigorous efforts to shape their work. It also indicates the differences and divisions among women workers, the varying conceptions that they have used to explain and defend their activities on the job. Professional leaders, the most visible of nurses, drew on the emerging conception of the career. They participated in the spirit of the first generation of college women, consciously turning from traditional commitment to the home to make paid work central to their lives. For these women, medical professionalization offered a model for the control over work and the public legitimacy they sought for nurses. In rebelling against the leaders, a few women looked back to nineteenth-century conceptions of duty, using religious and maternal imagery to describe the meaning of their work. As paid work gradually became more common and then typical for both married and single women, a third perspective grew stronger. Many, perhaps most, nurses took an intermediate stance between religious vocation and professional career to claim simply that nursing was their work, not their sacred duty or the center of their identity. All of these outlooks had a hand in forging nursing history; all tell us something about the opportunities and constraints that women confronted in their work and their lives.

In seeking to broaden nursing history's focus from professionalization to work experience, I realize that I have committed new sins of over-generalization and omission. My accounts of nurses on the job most often emphasize the common features of work and the solidarity fostered by shared experience; my discussion of conflict is generally confined to the troubled relationship of leaders with their rank and file. In fact, there were divisions, sometimes sharp divisions, among ordinary nurses too. Black women have always been underrepresented in nursing. Until the 1960s and sometimes later, they were relegated to separate and often inferior schools, limited to jobs in segregated wards, hospitals, or districts; they were denied military commissions even during the acute nursing shortage of World War II. Largely excluded from the American Nurses' Association, they formed their own active professional organization, the National Association for Colored Graduate Nurses. As hospitals slowly integrated, black nurses faced new forms of discrimination in hiring and struggled to claim the prerogatives of their skill against the entrenched expectations and prejudices of patients, doctors, and other nurses.[9] Ethnic and class differences among nurses are less visible in the records, but sometimes evident on the job. Foreign-born nurses often meet with resentment and ridicule. In nurses' informal work groups, the notoriously precarious position of nurses who are also doctors' wives is one vivid

example of class conflict. Marital status and sexual orientation
sometimes divide nurses on the job. Letters in the journals
indicate that married and single nurses have clashed, especially
in the 1940s and 1950s, as more and more married women
remained at work. In the workplace, gay nurses are sometimes
excluded from the sociability and camaraderie of the ward.
Finally, male nurses have their own story, one which illuminates questions of work and gender from another angle. Acknowledging this diversity and conflict within nursing, I have
nonetheless chosen to stress the common experiences of
nurses on the job.

Similarly, I have portrayed nursing leaders in broad
strokes, obscuring their differences and individual contributions to emphasize the professional ideology that they shared.
Many other sources fill this gap in my account. Nurses' own
histories, often overlooked except by nurses themselves, provide well-documented and insightful narratives of the professional associations and the women most active in them.

One use of language requires explanation. Because most
nurses have been women and most physicians men, I use
"nurse" as a feminine generic and "doctor" as a masculine
generic. As a feminist I eschew such usage in everyday life.
But as a feminist historian I have chosen these markers to
emphasize the sex-segregation of the work force in medicine
and nursing and to underscore my arguments about the relationship of gender and work.

"The Physician's Hand" traces nursing history from the
1920s to the 1970s. It begins just after World War I, at the peak
of the hospital schools' expansion. The "trained nurse" had
gained a secure place in medical care, but not yet found her
niche in the hospital; most nurses worked in private duty. As
that loosely organized freelance practice yielded to rationalized public health and hospital care, nurses faced dramatically
different problems and opportunities. This narrative explores
the changing social contexts of nursing care and the diverse
responses of leaders and nurses on the job. Chapter 1, "Not

Merely a Profession," outlines the theoretical framework of professionalization, its implications for nursing history, and its ultimate limitations as an interpretation of work, especially women's work. Chapter 2, "A Charge to Keep," examines the history and culture of the hospital schools, where young nurses underwent their apprenticeships and initiation into work. The following chapters focus on the changing structure and experience of nursing in its three major settings. Chapter 3, "The Freelance Nurse," portrays private-duty nurses at a moment of crisis, as the changing market of the 1920s and 1930s fractured the fragile advantages of freelance work. Chapter 4, "Public-Health Nurses and the 'Gospel of Health,'" explores the unusual autonomy of nurses associated with the crusade for preventive care from 1920 to 1950. The last chapter, "On the Ward," analyzes the transition from freelance to institutional work in the 1930s and its implications for nurses' practice in the next four decades. The Conclusion weighs the competing traditions of professionalization and occupational culture in nurses' history and their meaning for the current crisis in nursing.

CHAPTER 1

"Not Merely a Profession"

Writers on the professions have set forth conflicting definitions and interpretations, but all acknowledge the special place that professions occupy in the world of work. Common usages reveal the near-mystique associated with the concepts of professions and professionals. When we comment that someone is "a real professional," we bestow high praise: we mean an expert, someone fully qualified to perform the task at hand, one who can be trusted to assess and act on important problems. Professionals are their own bosses, not subject to the same close discipline as most workers. They occupy a special place in their communities: they are well paid, come home with clean hands, live in the best part of town. While others punch out at the end of the day, professionals carry their work identity into their private lives: friends and neighbors may even call them "Doc," "Judge," "Pastor," or "Professor," instead of their given names. Conversely, the label "unprofessional" is a weighty epithet, connoting haphazard, incompetent work; a casual, undignified approach to a serious matter; behavior that is unseemly, even morally suspect.

Nursing leaders, like members of many struggling occupations, have long sought to identify themselves with the prestige and the privileges of the professions. I have already suggested that they did not represent nursing's mainstream: the framework of professionalization can only encompass one part of a wider history. Moreover, I will argue here that it distorts that history, for nursing is not and cannot be a profession. My interpretation begins with a revisionist critique of the concept of professionalization, a perspective that dispels the mystique of the professions to present a more critical account of their structure and functions. This chapter then tests and extends that critique by applying it to the case of nursing. As an occupation seeking professional prerogatives, nursing offers a perspective on the social process of professionalization. As women's work, it illuminates the assumptions about gender that are built into professional ideology. Finally, I assess the impact of professional ideology on nursing, explicating the critical view of nursing leaders presented throughout *"The Physician's Hand."* As a strategy for nursing, professionalization is doomed to fail; as an ideology, professionalism divides nurses and weds its proponents to limiting and ultimately self-defeating values.

Many sociological and historical analyses of the professions simply confirm and elaborate upon the assumptions about professions that are revealed in everyday usage. Because they evoke these commonplace assumptions and because they have dominated the scholarly literature as well, I call them conventional or consensus interpretations. These accounts portray professions as the legitimate domains of expertise. Their members have extended theoretical knowledge in a body of esoteric and highly prized knowledge. They share a special altruism or commitment to service. Consensus interpretations acknowledge the professional's unusual autonomy in work and present this independence as appropriate, even essential. Possessors of special knowledge, professionals alone are fully equipped to judge and direct its application. The profession's clientele can grant this broad license with confidence because of the altruism that distinguishes the profession from ordinary callings. Released from most external supervision, professionals develop their own codes of ethics to ensure the responsible use of their knowledge. Members of professions set up mechanisms of peer review designed to monitor and regulate their practice. In addition, professionals carefully control access to their special privileges, setting standards for the education and certification of new practitioners to guarantee their competence and worthiness. Some observers also emphasize professionals' special orientation to work. Not only do they perform their duties with unusual altruism, but they also identify strongly with work, making it a part of their personalities in a way that workers in more mundane jobs increasingly resist.[1]

Critics of the conventional model have complained of its vague parameters, arguing persuasively that the definition does not provide meaningful distinctions among occupations. How long is "extended" training? How abstruse is "esoteric" knowledge? What are the boundaries between apprenticeship and theoretical education? How can we judge a profession's commitment to service in any objective way? Calling for a historical approach to the rise of the professions, one critic dismissed the consensus interpretation as "the sociologist's decoy" and pointed to its conservative implications. This formulation assumes that hierarchical organization of knowledge is necessary and desirable, and that a profession's power is derived primarily from the support of a broad social consensus. Accepting professionals' descriptions of their work at face value, sociologists (and historians) have ended by legitimating the professions rather than critically examining their structure and functions. As such, the conventional account is itself an example of professional ideology, not a definition of professions.[2]

Revisionists have turned from lists of attributes to broader structural and historical descriptions of the professions. Sociologist Eliot Freidson, an early advocate of this approach, argued that the defining characteristic of a profession is autonomy, professionals' unusual independence in defining the scope and application of their expertise. His analysis emphasizes the special character and power of this license. Professionals seek very broad social prerogatives. In medicine, for example, physicians claim not only the exclusive right to diagnose and treat illness, but also the right to control the division of labor in health services, to regulate related goods and services (such as the pharmaceutical industry), and even to name and control the social experiences of sickness and health.[3]

In accounting for the privileged position of the professions, revisionist formulations point to social power. While the conventional model asserts that professions win autonomy through their special expertise and their humanitarian concern for their clientele, critics have argued that members of a profession claim their dominant position with the support of a sponsoring elite. For medicine, revisionists have traced the role of nineteenth-century philanthropic foundations in reshaping and empowering the American medical profession. In this view, commitment to service does not define which occupations become professions; instead, a claim to altruism serves to legitimate professional prerogatives after the fact. Professionals are no more or less disinterested than any other workers, but because they claim power in such areas of intense cultural concern as sickness and health, they must justify their control and reassure their anxious clientele by seeming altruistic. Professional dominance is won through the agency of social elites, but maintained at least partly through the broader legitimacy provided by a trusting clientele. In this context, the ethical codes associated with professions take on a special ideological importance: they help to justify professional autonomy by manifesting the profession's commitment to service and providing the appearance of conscientious self-regulation.[4]

No profession has ever exercised the exclusive control or unconstrained autonomy that Freidson sees as a defining characteristic. A historical view modifies his structural description. Physicians won their professional privileges only after a long and contested struggle. They have seen corners of their empire eroded by the competing claims of other medical practitioners, and they have lost many of their battles for control to the active and powerful forces of third-party funding and the state. Finally, they maintain their commanding position at least partly at the sufferance of a public clientele that periodically rebels and challenges the legitimacy of professional expertise.

But if a revisionist model overstates the extent of medical dominance, it nonetheless provides an accurate description of the relative power that physicians exercise. Critics of the conventional model define professions in a way that makes sharper distinctions among occupations and emphasizes the controlling position of professions in a hierarchical division of labor. This structural analysis helps to locate nurses as workers. Clearly, nurses never gained the large measure of control over their work that defines a profession. The relationship between doctors and nurses in itself poses an intractable obstacle to nursing's professionalization. If professions maintain their authority through controlling the division of labor related to their work, as Freidson has argued, then doctors' own professionalization organizes and requires nurses' subordination.

This hierarchical relationship has not been static or absolute. The meaning and exercise of doctors' professional prerogatives have changed considerably over time. The different settings of medical care have also changed doctors' and nurses' relationships. On the job, nurses have developed complex ways of negotiating, interpreting, and revising their formal relationship. Nurses have seldom, if ever, simply carried out medical directives unthinkingly and automatically: they have always been more than "the physician's hand." But the medical hierarchy ultimately defines the boundaries of this variation. Doctors have consistently maintained and exercised the prerogative to define the scope of their own practice, and in so doing, they have claimed the right to set the limits of nurses' work.

Revisionist models of the professions have directed us to look beyond the structure of work to the social location of workers. Countering the consensus model's suggestion that professionals enjoy high social status because they do prestigious work, revisionists have asserted that professional work is prestigious partly because it is done by members of dominant social elites. Histories of successful professionalization indirectly support this argument by showing that efforts to upgrade work usually include upgrading the workers. In the reorganization of medical education, the effort to remove "irregular" practitioners also handily dispensed with disproportionate numbers of socially marginal practitioners: black, immigrant, and white working-class men and women from even the upper class. One can contest the direction of cause and effect in this example, but cases of other aspiring occupations indicate at least that would-be professionals try to upgrade work by bringing in socially superior workers. In nursing, leaders explicitly called for recruitment of "a higher class of young woman," and at various points in nursing history, others suggested recruiting men as a way to raise wages and win more respect for nursing. This interpretation recasts the significance of professions, suggesting that professions are not just special organizations of work but rather particular expressions and vehicles of dominant class and culture.

Women's history adds the analysis of gender to an explanation that has primarily emphasized class. Because women are the "second sex," I would argue, there can be no women's profession. We can identify female members of professions, but even our ways of speaking about them betray the anomaly of women in these positions: we mark their exceptional character by referring to a "woman doctor," a "woman lawyer," even, as I was once introduced, a "lady professor." Representing the most desirable work that our society offers, professional status is reserved for the most privileged. With few exceptions, white men from upper middle-class backgrounds fill the professions. Within the existing division of labor, nursing is not a profession, because nurses' autonomy is constrained by medicine's professional dominance. In broader cultural terms, nursing by definition cannot be a profession because most nurses are women.

Revisionist models have added depth and dimension to the conventional interpretation, but most retain a static quality. Historical interpretations of aspiring professions might sharpen and qualify the revised account. First, because of their focus on successful professions, critics may have underestimated the significance of professional ideology. Special knowledge and dedication to service do not in themselves confer professional privileges, but without a credible claim to them, no occupation can easily maintain the cultural legitimacy that supports the exercise of professional prerogatives. In established professions, such claims are more muted, tacitly understood, and accepted. Despite sharp public criticism and consumer rebellions in the last ten years, doctors still enjoy a large measure of public confidence and respect. A few might choose laetrile over conventional chemotherapy, home birth and self-help over hospital care, but no one questions physicians' special competence to perform a wide range of services, from prescribing drugs to transplanting organs. Established professions must polish up their images periodically; in upwardly mobile occupations, the appearance of competence and altruism becomes a more serious preoccupation. Whatever else they do, aspiring professionals try to define and expand the area of their legitimate expertise as they strive to persuade others of their devotion to public service.[5]

Moreover, studies of professionalization in process add a new perspective to the revisionist argument about social power and professional prerogatives. Aspiring professionals and their sponsors must fight for dominance on two fronts, overcoming external obstacles but also overpowering dissidents in their own ranks. Resistance to professionalization is not unique to nurses or to women workers. Historians of medicine have documented the protracted internal conflicts that accompanied the reorganization of medicine. Because of the character of professionalization, such opposition may well be virtually universal. The process draws clearer and tighter boundaries around an occupation. Autonomy is a privilege reserved to a select few, who gain the prerogative partly by dissociating themselves from their less presentable colleagues. An elite within the occupation establishes and defends control on higher ground, instituting educational reform or more rigorous certification requirements to restrict access to the profession. These freshly imposed standards inevitably exclude some of those already practicing, who are likely to resent this assault on their legitimacy and their livelihoods. This conflict clarifies the social relations that inform the division of labor, indicating the elitist and exclusionary character of professionalization.

The internal conflict in nursing reveals another dimension of the cultural meaning of professional ideology, its different implications for women.[6] Constructed by white male elites, the professions embodied an organization and an ideal of work derived from male experience. The leaders' strongest contribution, perhaps, lay in their claim to extend the privileges of a profession to women workers. In the process, they had to modify and reinterpret professional ideology to suit the conditions of women's work and to accommodate the social position of women workers.

Among the many nurses who resisted professionalization, a persistent minority attacked leaders as unwomanly. Standing outside the mystique of the professions, they criticized leaders for *downgrading* nurses' work by seeking professional prerogatives. These women interpreted professionalization in the context of traditional cultural values and expectations for women, and, in the process, they inadvertently revealed the gender specificity of professional ideology. Their viewpoint, which I call "traditionalist," centers on the premise that female character itself is the essential qualification for nursing. Strongest in the nineteenth century, this rhetoric flourished in a cultural and historical milieu that proclaimed female difference and moral superiority. Over the twentieth century, the notion of special fitness lost its force for most nurses, doctors, and laypersons, though it never disappeared altogether.

Claims of special fitness have often been invoked to justify and legitimate the existing sexual division of labor, and in this way, they lend support to women's subordination at work. But nurses have also used this traditional ideology to challenge the hierarchical values of professionalization and to oppose the exclusionary strategies of their professional leaders. One such moment occurred in the 1920s, when nurses confronted the mounting private duty crisis described in Chapter 3. By the 1920s, a time of growing specialization, the traditionalists were already anachronisms. But their argument nonetheless was telling evidence of the cultural sources of professional ideology and its special meaning for women.

In a culture and an occupation where the "expert" was increasingly revered, the traditionalists defined the nurse's skills as moral and religious rather than technical. Surrounded by the growing consumer economy of the 1920s, situated in a culture where money was a critical measure of worth, they asserted the value of self-abnegation over the worldly standards of wages. By echoing the nineteenth-century ideology of womanly service, these nurses dramatized the distance between domestic traditions of nursing and the new celebration of expertise.

These dissenting nurses felt that professional values represented the erosion of nursing's traditional commitment to service. They used the word "profession" to denote paid work, and associated it with narrow and self-seeking ambitions. "There are some who will maintain that nursing is merely a profession," one nurse acknowledged, "but there are others, many others, who were actuated by higher motives."[7] Another wrote: "Nursing is not merely a profession—it is a vocation; not merely a gainful occupation, but a ministry."[8] The professions claimed that a commitment to altruistic service distinguished them from the ordinary paid (men's) occupations. The formulation in itself revealed much about the growing instrumentality and alienation of work by the early twentieth century.[9] But these nurses spoke from outside the dominant culture to reverse the equation: for them, the word "profession" evoked the venal, secular spirit of paid work, exceptions to which existed only in the realm of the religious.

The traditional view again conflicted with the emerging

professional ideology in its conception of skill. Professional leaders touted the invaluable expertise that the trained nurse could bring to her practice and tirelessly promoted that skill to medical colleagues and lay constituencies. But in the moral and religious identity of the traditional nurse, technical expertise was carefully subordinated to a larger vision and mission. An 1889 graduate wrote, "We . . . feel that we give something more than mere skill to our service; we feel that we are expressing a broad humanitarian sentiment individualized."[10] While professional leaders worked to establish uniform and objective standards in nursing practice, traditionalists defended womanly empathy and intuition as nursing methods. As one nurse explained, "I always say to myself, 'How would the person who loves this patient the most try to work out this particular problem I am solving?"[11] In this conception of nursing, character and dedication were the real measures of a good nurse. Another wrote, "This work requires not only a skilled knowledge and expert training, but an aptitude—a talent—a love for a work where all thought of self must vanish and the whole man [sic] be given over to the care and cure of others."[12]

Professional ideology invested expertise with a kind of moral quality. It paired esoteric knowledge with altruism as defining attributes of the true profession, an association that implicitly suggested that experts deserved the special privileges of professional work. In contrast, traditionalists considered expertise as amoral at best. Their language betrayed an uneasiness about technical skill, a troubled sense that formal virtuosity, "mere skill," might overshadow nursing's humanitarian impulses. The professional concept of service essentially required no more than competent performance; its altruism was general and abstract, a vague commitment to a disembodied "public interest." The traditionalists' vision involved an intense, personal commitment, "a humanitarian sentiment individualized." This conception pressed the notion of service beyond professional responsibility to an ideal of religious abnegation. Traditionalists looked to the selfless woman, the nurturing mother—not to the expert.

The traditional connotations of womanly service confounded the leaders' claims to professional altruism. Men in an aspiring profession had to declare their special commitment to service, reflecting the larger assumption that paid work is instrumental and self-serving in nature. But as professional leaders strove to distinguish their work from women's unpaid domestic nursing, they had to dissociate themselves from the sentimental conception of womanly service. Thus the service component of professional ideology held different implications for men and women. Men, to establish their professional legitimacy, had to assert a stronger claim to service; women, to achieve the same end, had to escape the diffuse notion of womanly service.

This twist naturally created a quandary for those committed to a professional conception of work, since they could scarcely join battle against womanly virtue, motherhood, and Christian love. In more subtle ways, though, they did try to establish a distinction between the two conceptions of service. The journals contained both ideologies, but by the 1920s their editorials also illustrated the movement towards the more secular conception of nursing. The language of the traditionalists suggests that they felt themselves on the defensive, vainly shoring up an older position against the overwhelming tides of modern life. Lamenting the contemporary spirit, they asked, "Has the Nursing Instinct Died Out?" and "Is Religion in Our Schools Being Relinquished?"[13] Some blamed the distractions of a growing consumer society; one "pioneer nurse" explained that "in the past we had no telephones, no automobiles, and no picture shows to lure the young away from the straight and narrow," and deplored "the advancement of the ever-present world of Money Mad."[14] One nurse called for "a reawakening, a real religion, a reconsecration." A series of letters to the *American Journal of Nursing* (*AJN*) elaborated the same theme. In pondering the profession's problems, one writer noted with disapproval that two out of three nurses did not attend church regularly. She prescribed one hour a week in worship as the cure for nurses' difficulties, and somberly

warned the American Nurses' Association, "Any organization that rejects Jesus Christ will never grow!" This theme
continued in the letters column for several months; the last
exhorted, "Those who are not Christian people—wake up!"
But in a revealing rejoinder, *AJN* abruptly terminated the
debate with an icy editorial note: "We cannot continue this
correspondence."[15]

Elsewhere, professionally minded nurses explicitly dis-
claimed the sentimental vision of service and instead stressed
the nurse's technical expertise. One writer suggested, "Nurses
would perhaps prefer to have the 'angel of mercy' idea replaced by wording which would more carefully define the
physical, intellectual, and moral fitness of the true nurse to
work for community betterment."[16] This view of service con-
formed to the abstract public good of professional ideology,
not the religious commitment of the true woman. In strikingly similar terms, another wrote, "It is unfortunate and
harmful that nurses are so often called 'Angel of Mercy' instead of honest, painstaking workers. . . . They should be told
that they are fortunate in ranking among the workers of the
world and that there could be no better rank."[17] With rhetoric
like this, nurses disengaged from female domestic ideology
and embraced the values associated with paid work.

Finally, nurses confronted the professional conception of
work from their social position as women. For men, professional work represented mastery over skill and a vision of
unalienated work: not just a job, but a career. In a society
where men comprised most of the paid work force, and where
cultural expectations dictated paid work as man's duty, the
idea of a career embodied the most positive version of this
male experience. At a time when public life and private life
were increasingly perceived as separate domains, professional
ideology asserted their unity. A career blurred the line between work and private life, calling for intense personal identification with work and recreating work as the appropriate
domain of self-expression and self-fulfillment.

This formulation posed two thorny difficulties for aspiring female professionals. First, like the professional view of service, the concept of a career clearly distinguished the privileges of professions from the harsher conditions of most men's work. But in the context of women's traditional work at home, the idea of personal involvement in work threatened to translate itself from self-fulfillment back into the familiar terms of female self-sacrifice. Second, the professional emphasis on a career posed an intractable cultural contradiction for women, who were otherwise enjoined to make family and private life their primary commitment. For men, careers represented unalienated work, the rejoining of work and private life. For women, careers introduced a sharper conflict between the two realms. In the domestic ideal, a woman's work *was* private life. A woman who chose to invest much of her identity in paid work took the risk of cutting herself off altogether from the supports of marriage and family. For men, professional careers unambiguously embodied all that was most valued in work and public life: authority, self-control, skill, self-fulfillment. For women, careers symbolized the powerful contradiction of female experience itself. Being members of the same culture as men, they sometimes responded to the compelling attractions of careers in the same way; but as women they discovered, often at considerable social and emotional cost, that the rules and rewards of work were not the same for them.

The traditional view of nursing perhaps represented one response to these contradictory claims on women's lives. By emphasizing the noble mission of the nurse, one could reconcile commitment to paid work with cultural expectations for womanly service. Writing in this vein, some nurses urged self-abnegation with such zest that one suspects they were inspired by more than the glory of martyrdom. One contributor to *AJN* exalted the nurse as "a guardian of life . . . with her face ever toward the right and with a heart full of courage she is faithful to the end, ever conscious that there is one privilege, a greater blessing than receiving, and that is the pleasure of giving a life of service."[18] While one cannot discount the

power of such an ideology to motivate and reward its proponents, it also seems possible that this zeal was a coded expression of the self-fulfillment to be found in work.

Whatever its covert meaning, however, this sentimental
expression grated on nurses who were committed to professional ideology. In rejecting the "angel of mercy" image,
some nurses also directly addressed and challenged its conception of female self-abnegation. "Isn't it rather a *realization of
self* than a *sacrifice of self* to be able to do worthwhile necessary
work which calls forth all of our resources for its adequate
performance, and challenges us to add continuously to those
resources? Surely such a service is no sacrifice."[19] Such a notion
represented a radical innovation for women. With it leaders
defended women's entitlement to work for its own sake, an
idea that women are still struggling to assert against longstanding and deeply entrenched opposition.

If nursing is not and cannot be a profession, what was the
meaning of the leaders' preoccupation with professional ideology? Although nurses never achieved the prerogatives of professionals, the struggle for that status influenced the direction
of nursing history. The leaders' uncritical acceptance of professional ideology was both a source of strength and a serious
weakness. On the one hand, professional aspirations empowered nurses, pushing them beyond the confines of domestic
ideology into the new possibilities of the labor market. Leaders brought a certain realism and vitality to the problems of
nursing, measuring nurses' positions by the standards and
values of the world of paid work, not the lost world of an
idealized domesticity. In identifying themselves with professionals, they tried to act as men's equals in the world of paid
work. They refused the limiting conventions of gender in
their own lives and in their goals for nursing as an occupation.
Although most nursing leaders did not identify themselves as
feminists, their commitment to work and their efforts to claim
professional privileges did implicitly challenge and unsettle
traditional constraints on women in the workforce.

But their professional aspirations proved both unproductive and divisive. Adopting the exclusionary tactics of professionalization, leaders sought to secure the privileges of a few at the expense of many. As women they could not hope to win the privileges of a profession, and as aspiring professionals they cut themselves off from the broader support that a more inclusive program could have provided; they eschewed other occupational strategies, such as trade unionism, that might have proved more effective. Finally, they committed themselves to a self-defeating ideology. To the extent that the leaders endorsed a professional hierarchy based on expertise, they participated in maintaining their own subordination. Within the logic of professionalization, doctors had an unshakeable claim to the controlling position in the medical division of labor: they could be unseated only by a direct challenge to the values of professional ideology.

Professional ideology shaped and limited leaders' activities throughout the history of organized nursing. Following the lead of physicians, lawyers, teachers, and others in the late nineteenth century, prominent nurses sought to reorganize and regulate occupational certification and practice. Reform in nursing was commonly identified with Florence Nightingale's renowned work in English hospitals, and indeed, American nursing leaders did shape their own educational goals with an eye to Nightingale's ideals and achievements. As important, they worked to join nursing to a broader transformation occurring in other occupations by the 1870s. As nursing leaders established the first generation of hospital schools between 1873 and 1893, they committed themselves to the assumptions and strategies of professionalization. They used professional ideology to defend nursing as paid work, distinguishing it from the diffuse category of women's domestic duty. But they also invoked professional ideology to preserve this new occupation for an elite group of women.

Every nursing history acknowledges the influence of Florence Nightingale, and so must this one. Firmly in the tradition of Victorian reform, Nightingale struggled to improve English hospitals through the uplifting influence of genteel women. She recruited upper-class women to supervise their disreputable sisters and introduced regular routines and military discipline into the casual disorder of nineteenth-century hospital life. Inspired by Nightingale's example, reform-minded women in the United States began to investigate and reorganize the care in their own charitable hospitals. In 1873, the first three training schools opened at Bellevue Hospital in New York, Massachusetts General Hospital in Boston, and Connecticut Hospital in New Haven. The idea of a training course for nurses spread slowly, and "trained nurses," the graduates of these early hospital courses, were a rarity. In 1880, an estimated 560 of them were scattered among the 13,000 "practical nurses" listed in the United States census. In 1890, only 35 schools were operating.[20]

Nevertheless, the first generation of American nursing superintendents successfully transformed the social environment of those hospitals that had nursing schools. In 1881, the superintendent of Boston City Hospital surveyed her students with satisfaction, noting, "I was very happy to notice a higher type of womanhood represented. . . . "[21] Dispelling the air of disrepute that clung to the untrained nursing attendants who had staffed earlier hospitals, the new breed of nurses also subdued remaining elements of hospital low life. One of the lay board members of the Bellevue Training School reported the ennobling influence of refined women. Anxious not to offend them, doctors began to provide screens for their patients on the wards. Even medical students, a notoriously unruly group, curbed their boisterous behavior in deference to the ladies.[22] Student nurses themselves jealously guarded their reputations. A nurse who entered the Pittsburgh Training School in 1893 commented on other students' consciousness of breeding and "background," recalling their scorn for a new classmate, "a big raw-boned country girl from somewhere upstate."[23] Nursing students' prior education suggested the class base of this gentility. In the 1890s, 32 percent of the students in training schools had graduated from high school, as compared to only 2 percent of young women in the whole population.[24]

Between 1890 and 1920, broad changes in medical care created unprecedented opportunities for the trained nurse. Scientific advances and other social changes supported the development of nursing as skilled paid labor. When Nightingale published *Notes on Nursing* in 1860, nursing care was part of women's household responsibilities. Her manual itself signaled the changing character of care: womanly instinct, she warned, was not enough for skilled nursing. But she directed her advice to laywomen, offering common-sense instruction on the arts of home nursing. By the 1920s, new medical knowledge had placed nursing skills on a more scientific basis. In treatment of contagious diseases, for example, precise isolation techniques based on the germ theory replaced the general principles of good housekeeping that had served Nightingale's nurses. Other social changes also influenced the laywoman's displacement by a paid nurse. Some historians have suggested that newly isolated middle-class families began to hire private-duty nurses for home care and to resort more often to hospital care as urban life disrupted the old resources of extended families. This combination of scientific and social change reinforced the training schools' efforts to distinguish between the trained nurse and traditional lay nurses.[25]

Finally, by the late nineteenth century, medical practice was shifting from patients' homes to hospitals. As the techniques of antisepsis and asepsis became widely accepted and used, hospitals could offer new therapies and safer care. With more reliable asepsis, the terrible post-surgical mortality rates of the early nineteenth century fell, and surgical intervention increased dramatically. Offering new opportunities to medical practitioners, hospitals became laboratories for experimental techniques, treatments, and research. Patient care improved with knowledge of the causes and transmission of contagious disease: isolation techniques helped to confine infections that had once swept through the wards. Hospitals drew more private physicians and attracted a growing middle-class clientele. Once scarce and widely scattered, hospitals became a commonplace feature of urban and suburban landscapes. In 1873, when the first nursing schools were founded, there were fewer than 200 hospitals in the United States. By 1910, over 4,000 were open, and less than two decades later, 7,416 were offering their services. From the charitable institutions of Nightingale's day, hospitals were becoming centers for a prestigious and profitable service industry.[26]

Hospital expansion provided the economic motivation and base for the establishment of hundreds of new training schools for nurses. Nursing schools opened all over the country as flourishing hospitals sought a more disciplined workforce and as administrators wooed a fee-paying clientele by replacing attendants with respectable student nurses. The reforms that Nightingale and others had instituted earlier had produced a worker that neatly suited these requirements. Indeed, some historians have suggested that earlier hospital reform in itself had accelerated the use of the hospital. Observing the new order that trained nurses brought to hospital wards, doctors may have brought middle-class patients to hospitals more readily. In any case, after 1890 training courses multiplied along with hospitals. By 1910, one in four hospitals had nursing schools, and in 1927, 2,155 hospital schools kept their wards supplied with student nurses.[27]

Nursing leaders observed this burgeoning growth with decidedly mixed emotions. On the one hand, it was gratifying confirmation of their claims for the superiority of the trained nurse. Doctors and laypersons alike had often challenged the idea of nursing education, content with older conceptions of nursing as a domestic art. Although some die-hards still scoffed, by World War I nursing was widely accepted as the province of experts. Wartime shortages and the ravages of influenza brought a vocal public demand for more trained nurses. However, as the cause of the trained nurse gained legitimacy, leaders lost control over the management and mission of the schools. No longer were new programs established on their initiative or under their careful guidance. Nightingale's American counterparts had set up hospital schools to demonstrate the value of a trained worker. Hospital administrators seized on a rather different possibility: they saw student nurses as a permanent source of labor. Eager to capitalize on this new resource, they opened their own schools, offering maintenance and a training course in exchange for two or three years of ward service. The graduates went on to private duty, and superintendents recruited new crops of students for hospital work. The *American Journal of Nursing* frequently deplored the renegades in their own ranks who facilitated this wild growth, those trained nurses who went to work as hospital superintendents and set up schools that did not conform to the Nightingale ideal.[28]

Professional associations were organized at least partly in response to the uncontrolled expansion of hospital schools. In them, nurses worked to set uniform standards, protecting their own credentials against dilution by the outpouring of graduates from questionable schools. Women trained in the older schools constituted a self-conscious elite, separating themselves from the students and superintendents associated with the younger hospital schools. In 1893, a few leaders organized the American Society of Superintendents of Training Schools (ASSTS), composed of carefully selected superintendents of the larger schools in the United States and Canada. The same schools began to form alumnae associations in 1888, and in 1896, the Nurses' Associated Alumnae (NAA) provided a national organization to link the local networks of the schools. Like the ASSTS, the group selected its membership, excluding alumnae organizations from smaller or narrowly specialized hospitals. Both groups worked to establish firmer educational standards. The NAA also organized state registration campaigns to ratify and enforce minimum standards of preparation.[29]

In the next decade, the associations reorganized and sought a broader membership. In 1900, the Nurses' Associated Alumnae began to publish the *American Journal of Nursing*.

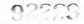

A few years later, the groups split into separate organizations in the United States and Canada. In 1911, the Nurses' Associated Alumnae dissolved to form again as the American Nurses' Association and the Canadian Nurses' Association, and membership was extended to all graduate nurses from approved schools. The next year, the National League of Nursing Education took over the functions of the old ASSTS, and, like the ANA, extended its membership somewhat.

Despite their attempts to organize on a wider basis, the associations retained the assumptions and goals of their founding elites. Their reform efforts were far-sighted in conception but narrowly based, directed at protecting a minority within nursing. Leaders in the associations had correctly identified many of the problems that nursing faced as an occupation. The apprenticeship system could be harshly exploitative, and the varying standards of the schools left patients vulnerable to incompetent care. But the solutions leaders offered reflected an underlying concern with preserving the prerogatives of an elite group of better-educated nurses. By stiffening educational standards, they struggled to recover the elite position of early training schools. In 1898, at a time when most nurses had not graduated from high school and few hospitals hired full-time instructors, the ASSTS had already begun to press for college-educated nurses in supervisory and training positions. The leaders of this generation—Adelaide Nutting, Isabel Maitland Stewart, Lillian Wald, Isabel Hampton Robb, Lavinia Dock—were all firmly committed to collegiate education for nurses. Over the twentieth century, the NLNE and the ANA would cling to this emphasis on credentials, remaining somewhat removed from the immediate problems of nurses on the job.

At bottom, leaders and other nurses faced the expansion between 1890 and 1920 from fundamentally different positions. Most nurses experienced the sharply rising demand for their services as a new opportunity. A new category of paid work had opened up at a time when working women faced limited choices, especially for white-collar jobs. Young women poured enthusiastically into the schools and then into the private-duty market. Those nurses who became hospital superintendents or administrators clearly had even stronger reasons for applauding the expansion of nursing. But for aspiring professionals, rising demand posed a threat as well as a potential opportunity. Committed to upgrading nursing as an occupation, leaders were unwilling to undertake the task of upgrading nurses already in practice. Rather than casting their lot with the growing number of nurses, leaders pursued the restrictive strategy of professionalization. The following chapters trace the consequences of that choice in nursing's persistent internal conflict, and outline the alternatives to professional ideology that nurses developed in the hospital schools and on the job.

CHAPTER 2

"A Charge to Keep": Hospital Schools of Nursing, 1920–1950

Nurses' distinctive training set them aside from other working women and formed the core of their occupational culture. Until the 1950s, virtually every school required that the student nurse live in the hospital's nursing residence, so the hospital was school, workplace, and home combined. Separated from her family and community, the young woman took her place in a world of female authority, where she underwent a rigorous apprenticeship into nursing, learning her craft in classrooms and on the ward. Within a few months—sometimes within hours—the new student would venture into the ward, first arranging flowers or scrubbing utensils, then gradually advancing to tasks that demanded more skill and knowledge. Superintendents drilled and disciplined her, constantly reminding her of her special mission and grave responsibilities. Hard work, strict discipline, and the shocks of hospital life bonded students together and initiated them into a common occupational identity.

Nursing histories often portray the hospital school as an unfortunate historical accident, a product of the imperatives of hospital expansion, rather than of nurses' own needs and goals. Certainly the schools had close economic ties with the hospitals; they drew funding from the hospital budget, and students provided most of the nursing services. Through the 1920s, most hospitals with schools depended entirely on student nurses, hiring graduate nurses only for a few supervisory positions. While hospitals began to hire some graduates for ward duty in the 1930s, student nurses continued to work in both staff and supervisory positions into the 1950s. But nurses were not merely the hapless victims of this system. Indeed, some nurses actively perpetuated it as hospital superintendents and administrators, and many more affirmed its methods and values. The schools represented a coherent ideology of their own that offered a powerful alternative, and sometimes a direct challenge, to the values of professional ideology.

The schools stood at the center of the conflict between professional leaders and other nurses. While the content and conduct of nurses' training changed between 1920 and 1950, the debate remained remarkably consistent in that period, reflecting the persistent ideologies and traditions of each group. For those committed to professionalization, educational reform represented a key strategy. Beginning with a 1912 survey, prominent nurses railed against apprenticeship training. Critical of the wide variation in the schools' programs, they pressed for uniform requirements for admission, standard curriculums, and a program weighted toward academic education rather than ward experience. In the professional associations, leaders struggled to establish and control accrediting of the schools. Committed to professional autonomy, they also sought to separate nursing education from hospital ward service. Leaders called for graduate hospital staffs to release students from the responsibility of running the nursing service, and they argued that students should pay tuition rather than receive stipends. Throughout, they stressed the value of a "professional" education—that is, a program oriented to theoretical knowledge, based in colleges and universities rather than in hospitals.

As the reformers often pointed out, many of the superintendents and graduates who defended the hospital schools had a strong material interest in the existing system. Hospital administrators, many of whom were nurses, were reluctant to pay graduates for services that students would perform in exchange for room, board, training, and a small stipend. Superintendents exercised considerable autonomy under the apprenticeship system, running their schools and their wards according to their own notions of proper training and discipline. "Professional" education, removed from the hospital, would drastically reduce their control. Many graduates resisted standardization of education and practice, defending themselves against an upgrading that would devalue their own skills and their hospital school diplomas. Nurses' resistance to professionalization also drew on deep ideological differences. Skeptical of the claims of educational reformers, they upheld apprenticeship training as a part of nursing's craft tradition. In this conception, education meant more than acquiring skills and knowledge: it was a process of initiation that transformed the student from a laywoman into a nurse.

This chapter inverts the familiar history of progress in nursing education, told from the viewpoint of professional leaders, to reconsider the claims and experience of the losers, those nurses steeped in the apprenticeship tradition. The ideology and culture of the schools stood at the center of nursing history: the hospital programs provided a common experience shared by generations of practitioners. Until 1971, the diploma schools graduated more new nurses than associate and baccalaureate programs combined; even as late as 1974, 76 percent of all active nurses held diplomas from hospital schools.[1] Apprenticeship training ultimately outlived its usefulness, just as professional leaders had predicted. But it also had special strengths. In the schools, young women learned responsibility and commitment to work, and they were initiated into a distinctive craft culture.

I. IN PURSUIT OF PROFESSIONALIZATION

During the rapid expansion of nursing between 1890 and 1920, the surveys and analyses made by nursing leaders reflected a continuing lack of control over nursing education and practice. The professional associations lobbied hard for licensing to establish uniform standards and to control admission to nursing practice, with only limited success. By the mid-1920s, all the states had laws that acknowledged but did not enforce professional accrediting of nursing schools. Under this permissive legislation, graduates of accredited hospital schools could submit their diplomas to state boards and receive their stamp of approval along with the title "registered nurse." But graduates were not required to register, and, more important, other self-styled nurses were not legally restrained from practicing, so the laws had little effect on the education or employment of nurses. The first mandatory licensing law was not passed until 1938, in New York, and most laws remained weak until after World War II, with standards varying widely from state to state.[2]

Concerned with the rapid growth of nursing in this unregulated market, the American Nurses' Association established a committee to study the economics of nursing, and commissioned sociologist May Ayres Burgess to run an extensive survey of nursing education and practice. In 1928, the Burgess report, *Nurses, Patients, and Pocketbooks*, was published, providing a wealth of statistical and interview data. Comparing nursing and medical education between 1880 and 1926, the report revealed both the expectations and the frustrations of nurses who aspired to professional status. The number of medical schools had peaked in 1906, when 161 were open; even by then, 432 schools were producing nurses. By 1926, doctors had cut the number of medical schools in half, to 79. Meanwhile, hospital schools had increased more than fourfold: 2,155 institutions pumped out graduates.[3] The Burgess report underscored the growing oversupply of nurses and urged closer regulation of nursing education and practice.

Nursing was desperately in need of some such rationalization. As it was practiced in the 1920s, the apprenticeship system posed certain intractable limits to nurses' education and employment. As leaders argued constantly, hospital schools existed primarily to provide nursing service, and such an arrangement inevitably made students vulnerable to abuse. As the first official survey of hospital schools revealed in 1912, the academic arrangements of such schools were often informal at best; 315 schools, or nearly 45 percent, reported that they did not have a single paid instructor, and 299 did not maintain a library. Instead, the nursing "curriculum" in many hospitals consisted of two or three years of ward work. The value of such apprenticeships was uneven. In larger hospitals, students might benefit from a stimulating environment of medical innovation, and learn the nursing care of a wide variety of conditions. But many of the schools were located in small hospitals; in 1912, 60 percent of the schools were in institutions with a daily patient average of under 75, and 25 percent operated in hospitals that served fewer than 25 patients a day. In this setting, the student's practical experience might be curtailed by the limited services a small institution provided. Few hospitals had systematic plans for rotating students through their different services; rather, students worked where their hands were most needed and learned what they could there.[4]

By the mid-1920s, leaders also recognized that hospital schools were creating a severe employment crisis. Reluctant to hire graduate nurses for their regular ward service, hospitals replenished their workforces by recruiting new crops of students. The result was that, between 1900 and 1920, the number of trained nurses rose from 11,804 to 149,128, while the population of the United States increased by less than 50 percent.[5] Even in the context of rapidly increasing demand for medical and nursing services, this flood of new nurses could not be absorbed. A few graduates found supervisory jobs in hospitals, and still fewer moved into the small new field of public health. But most graduated from their training schools to work in the uncertain freelance market of private-duty nursing. Before World War I, there were already ominous signs of the collapse of the private-duty market, and by the 1920s many nurses were struggling desperately for work. Meanwhile, the hospitals cried out for more nurses and continued to recruit students.

Leaders identified these problems early through careful and detailed surveys, and argued eloquently for reform. In one sense, their professional aspirations gave them a breadth of vision: they had a perspective on the larger structure of the occupation that other nurses sometimes lacked. They shrewdly assessed the direction of nursing and medicine, predicting that hospitals would come to depend on graduate nurses and working to define their place to the best advantage. They believed in women's education and tried passionately to make nurses' training equal to the best of it. But as they looked to the future of nursing and strived to make their vision real, they seldom gave more than a backward glance to those who would be left behind. The victims of inferior schools, the respectable graduates without high school diplomas, the young women without the money for tuition in hospital schools or universities—all were to be sacrificed to the hope of professionalization.

Those who held professional goals looked askance at many of their new colleagues. Superintendents wrote to complain of their trying experiences in the schools, as hospital expansion and the constant demand for more student nurses forced more liberal standards of admission. Writing in 1926, one described the formidable problems of instructing girls who lacked "a background of culture" and "home training in the finer things," and implored, "Can we make bricks without straw?"[6] Another superintendent despaired of upholding standards in schools eager for student labor. She described the fates of twelve students she had dismissed "for many reasons, varying from poor scholarship to illegitimate pregnancy and coming into the dining room so drunk they vomited on the table." In spite of this disreputable behavior, the wicked had prospered. Ten of the offenders had been admitted to other schools and later graduated. The last two students, clearly incorrigibles, were admitted and then dismissed from a second school, but both gained admission at a third hospital and finally graduated. None of the schools had investigated the students' earlier records.[7] The Burgess report concluded grimly, "The willingness of some hospitals to admit young women of doubtful character and low intellectual capacity is so well known that in some places the public assumes that all nurses must be of that type."[8]

Between 1890 and 1920, many new hospitals opened and use of existing facilities increased. During World War I the demand for nurses became even more acute, and the influenza epidemic that followed created another outcry for nurses. Under such pressures, superintendents could not always hold out for well-bred ladies, and probably not all placed the same value on a young woman's background. As the nursing workforce grew, the genteel women of the first schools necessarily gave way to a less rarefied breed.[9]

Some sources indicate that elite nurses were responding, not to a dramatic degeneration in quality, but to a relative decline in nursing's status. The rapid spread of high school education and the expansion of women's white-collar work had revised the clearly elite position of the trained nurse of the 1890s. As one observer lamented, "Years ago, nurses were drawn from the best educated groups of their day. Now, in many cities, it requires more education to get a job as a shop girl than to enter a school of nursing. Many department stores are requiring high school graduation for salesgirls, as a matter of course. It is practically impossible to get a job as a stenographer in a good firm without being a high school graduate."[10] Yet in terms of educational qualifications, young nurses in the 1920s were actually superior to their 1890 counterparts. A 1928 survey reported that 56 percent of nurses were high school graduates, compared to 32 percent in the earlier generation. And as a group, student nurses in the 1920s were better educated than their non-nurse peers; more than half were high school graduates, compared to 30 percent of all young women.[11] If few nurses came from the most elite social circles, nursing probably still drew more heavily than other women's occupations from the middle class. Burgess's survey found that nurses' fathers were more likely than other men in their age group to work in professions and trades, and less likely to hold jobs in manufacturing, mining, and domestic services. While nurses were somewhat less likely than other women of their age to have native-born parents, most of the immigrant parents came from Canada and the British Isles, representing respectable Anglo-Saxon stock.[12]

Although legal standards for licensure remained low, nurses' educational qualifications continued to improve. A 1930 survey, for example, showed that, while only nine states required high school graduation for state registration, 71 percent of a random sample of student nurses were high school graduates. Two years later, another study indicated that 90 percent met this standard. Throughout the 1920s and 1930s, most schools apparently raised their requirements well above the low limits set by state registration laws. A 1934 report claimed, "Full high school education or its equivalent is now accepted as an almost universal requirement for entrance to the nursing profession."[13]

The character of nurses' training also began to change in the 1920s and 1930s, with classroom work gradually assuming more importance. Leaders had long urged schools to charge tuition rather than paying their students stipends, hoping that the income from tuition would replace some of the students' in-kind ward service. During the 1930s, many hospitals obliged by cutting the student allowance and charging tuition. In 1932, 88 percent of schools paid their students, while seven years later, only 38 percent provided a stipend.[14] More graduates were hired for general duty positions, lifting some of the burden from the nursing school. By the mid-1930s, students' hours on duty had decreased somewhat, as leaders had hoped, although in nearly three-quarters of the schools they still worked eight hours a day or more.[15] The *American Journal of Nursing* enthusiastically reported new studies and experiments that indicated that some schools were developing more structured curriculums. Practical work still dominated the training, but students attended classes for three to six months before working regular ward shifts, and they rotated through different services systematically, rather than shuttling around to fill in on the busiest floors.[16]

The national crises of depression and war pressed nursing toward the rationalization that leaders had sought. Strained by increased patient loads and slow payments during the depression years, hospitals began to question the economy of student services. Many of the smaller hospitals closed their schools, eliminating some of the programs most remote from leaders' standards.[17] Although graduates were still produced at an alarming rate, the number of schools dropped. By 1940, only 1,235 diploma schools were open, a considerable reduction from the 2,155 schools of 1928. The professional associations could look with pride to 76 additional institutions that offered baccalaureate education for nurses.[18] As hospitals turned to graduate staffing in the 1930s, employment problems lessened and then evaporated altogether in the scramble to secure nurses for war service.

World War II further accelerated the standardization process. Overnight, national mobilization of nurses gave the schools a common program. Funded by the federal government and designed in cooperation with the professional associations, the Cadet Nurse Corps offered favorable terms to qualifying hospitals and students. Hospitals had to have a daily patient average of fifty, cutting out the problematic smaller institutions at a stroke. Virtually all student nurses who trained in the war years belonged to the program, responding to patriotic rhetoric and the inducements of free training, uniforms, and books, plus a small stipend. All had to have records of good academic performance and high school diplomas, and all participated in an accelerated thirty-month program of theory and practice. Most worked an additional six-month stint on the ward to meet state requirements for three years of training.[19]

During World War II, nursing leaders moved decisively to increase the numbers of baccalaureate nurses and to establish more collegiate programs. A special committee worked to recruit women at five hundred colleges and universities for nurses' training, focusing attention on institutions of higher education rather than appealing to high school girls, the traditional audience for recruiters. In the National Nursing Council for War Service, the wartime coalition of all the professional associations in nursing, a committee assigned to "domestic postwar planning" discussed ways to set up training programs within universities.[20]

The outlines of today's nursing education and practice were visible by the end of the war. Nurses were initially concerned about the possibility of postwar glut like that of the 1920s, but it soon became clear that hospitals were a growth industry. Stimulated by new federal funding and expanding support from third-party sources (especially Blue Cross and Blue Shield insurance), hospital services boomed. With wartime medical and surgical advances, patient care grew more sophisticated, increasing nurses' skills and securing their places in the hospital. The informal division of labor that had always existed in the hospital began to harden. The old "attendants" became licensed practical nurses and nurses' aides, managed and supervised by registered nurses. R.N.s themselves became more minutely divided by skill and function as new specialties developed and as administration became more rationalized and complex.

The 1948 Brown report, *Nursing for the Future*, marked a critical divide in nursing history. Commissioned by the National Nursing Council, the report embodied the professional aspirations of nursing leaders and signaled the postwar intentions and direction of the professional associations. Written by Esther Lucile Brown of the Russell Sage Foundation, *Nursing for the Future* boldly asserted the goal of baccalaureate education for nurses. Since the late nineteenth century, aspiring professionals had emphasized the importance of university-based education; in this sense, the Brown report simply represented a continuity. But its final recommendations constituted an important turning point, for the report firmly removed the diploma schools from nursing's future.

In the conclusion, Brown conceded that hospital programs would remain open for a time as an "interim solution" to the urgent demand for nursing services, but she asserted that such programs would have no place in a fully reformed nursing education. Brown also ratified and extended the emerging division of labor in nursing, openly labeling the diploma graduate as a second-class citizen. The report proposed a new hierarchy within nursing, with the "professional" or baccalaureate nurse on top and the "technical" nurse or hospital graduate as her subordinate. Leaders had moved from a critique of hospital schools to a full-scale attack on apprenticeship training.[21]

The findings of the Brown report and subsequent efforts to implement it indicate the elite and divisive character of professionalization. The report documented the persistence of apprenticeship training. In 1947, diploma programs still emphasized clinical work after an initial six months in the classroom, and 88 percent of nurses had no college credits; nonetheless, leaders proposed to reserve the prized label of "professional" for the few degree-holding nurses.[22] The Committee to Implement the Brown Report plowed ahead with an accrediting system, endorsing only a small proportion of existing programs even under more tolerant "interim" standards. A 1951 assessment gave full approval to only 167 out of 1,060 hospital schools, rendering critical judgments on eight out of nine. Predictably, collegiate programs fared better, though many of these also failed the rigorous test of newly elevated standards; 51 out of 117 degree programs won full approval.[23] Once again leaders' "professional" standards set the limits of their alliances: they sought to reserve the best jobs—and the very title of professional nurse—for those nurses who could claim degrees. This time they would win, although it would take nearly thirty more years to close the hospital schools.

II. THE CULTURE OF APPRENTICESHIP

While by 1950 the defenders of traditional nursing education were beginning to lose the war, the Brown report itself showed that they still controlled the battleground. Hospital schools trained the overwhelming majority of nurses, and most of them inculcated their charges with a view of nursing that diverged rather sharply from leaders' visions. Apprenticeship stood at the center of the hospital school's method and mission. Although in part a managerial strategy, it was also an ideology of what nursing should be and a carefully articulated method for making young women into competent and committed nurses.

An early ethics manual advised that "to become a good trained nurse, development must come from three sides—the hands, the heart, and the head."[24] Defenders of the hospital schools heartily endorsed that sentiment and would have approved the order as well. They valued the craft skills of nursing—gentle hands, a deft injection, careful handling of the patient in pain. The cold objectivity of an academic degree was no fit measure of "the nursing heart," and classroom work could do little to nurture the qualities of an ideal nurse: "a sense of honor, a sense of humor, a sense of order, a humane heart, patience and self-control."[25] Superintendents of hospital schools confidently set out to mold their human material to these exacting requirements. For these women, nursing education was more than the mastery of a body of knowledge, it was a moral initiation: "The drilling and disciplining of the woman inside the nurse, the development of a right attitude of mind and right habits of life, are the most difficult as well as the most important part in the making of a nurse."[26]

These sweeping objectives were both the weakness and the strength of the hospital schools. Setting out "to shape the young nurse's total personality," superintendents could claim broad authority over students' lives, and very broad prerogatives for themselves. The paternalistic discipline of the hospital could be petty and arbitrary, alienating independent young women. At times, the defense of craft skills and empathy verged on anti-intellectualism: some nurses resisted the very notion of liberal education with unreasoning vehemence. Yet the same ideology provided nurses with strong preparation and motivation to work. Rooted deeply in the realities of the ward, hospital programs gave nurses a direct socialization into the work they would do as graduates. Moreover, the insularity of the schools and the intensity of hospital life comprised a powerful rite of passage. Separated from the claims of the larger culture, a bit distant from its prescriptions for women, nursing students might find new and compelling models for female commitment to work.

Manuals, oral and written memoirs, and fiction reveal the emotional impact of the student nurse's apprenticeship. Graduates from the 1920s and the 1950s retell their experiences of training in strikingly similar ways: common perceptions and values blur the actual historical differences in their educations. These are narratives of initiation, of a journey from innocence to knowledge. As they begin, the narrator is an outsider describing the initial strangeness and threat of the hospital world. The trials and rituals of ward duty challenge her, and gradually she learns the skills and discipline of a nurse. Once inept at ward duties, frightened or repelled by hospital life, the young nurse comes to master her responsibilities and take pride in her abilities. Advancing through the training course, she gains the perspective and privileges of the insider.

The special environment of the hospital shaped the student's experience of apprenticeship and initiation. Nursing schools fit Erving Goffman's classic definition of a "total institution," a place where the usual social boundaries between public and private life collapse. "Inmates" of total institutions sleep, work, and play under a single pervasive authority. Subordinated to this authority, they lose or surrender many of their normal prerogatives. Their most mundane activities are closely controlled; their most intimate actions are open to surveillance. Total institutions deliberately construct a separate social world, marked off by systematic and routine violations of "outside" expectations. While normal social rules balance individual autonomy against the demands of social life, total institutions submerge or deny individual claims in the service of institutional goals.[27]

Hospital superintendents maintained strict control over students' work and social lives, exercising an authority that extended well past the normal limits of school or workplace discipline. Student nurses had to live in the hospital nursing residence, cut off from familiar surroundings, family, and friends. Long working hours, early curfews, and prohibitions against socializing with male co-workers further constrained their social lives. The demands of ward duty, as interpreted by the superintendent, reigned over all other considerations. A student nurse had little time that she could call her own. Superiors arranged her ward hours and classroom schedules, determined her meal times and study hours, and governed her hours of sleep. On or off duty, her appearance and demeanor had to conform to rigid standards of propriety. At one training school in 1918, for example, students were not permitted to cut their hair; in the 1930s, another superintendent forbad bleached hair.[28] Supervisors inspected students' rooms and mustered their nurses before ward duty for inspection. One nurse remembered ruefully that everyone in the school was required to wear her uniform sixteen inches from the floor, regardless of her own height; the superintendent, a stickler for symmetry, wanted her students' hems to form an unbroken line when the group assembled.[29] Even the most intimate bodily functions might come under the superintendent's relentless scrutiny. In an extreme example, one article urged superintendents to record each student's menstrual periods, to provide "anti-constipation" diets, and to segregate "fat and lean" groups in the dining room, with appropriate foods for each.[30] Discipline, efficiency, and regularity could go no farther.

From her first days at school, the student nurse learned the elaborate rituals of hospital hierarchy. Advice manuals presented "hospital etiquette" as a symbol of respect for superiors and a sign of the nurse's own seriousness and responsibility. One description conveys the ceremonial quality of professional deference. "The head-nurse and her staff should stand to receive the visiting physician, and from the moment of his entrance until his departure, the attending nurses should show themselves alert, attentive, and courteous, like soldiers on duty."[31] In the same way, entering students deferred to their nursing superiors, including superintendents, directors, head nurses, instructors, and students in the upper classes. In the 1920s, seniority systems applied even within the first-year class: students were arbitrarily ranked in the order that they arrived at the training school.[32]

Goffman has described the use of mortification of the self for inducting new members into total institutions, and indeed probationers were reminded of their humble status many times a day. They had to stand for their innumerable superiors, follow them into elevators, open doors for them, line up behind them in the dining room. As one character in a nursing novel summarized, hospital etiquette "all boiled down to the creed that probationers were worms of the dust, and were to admit it at every possible opportunity."[33]

In accepting the rigid codes of hospital hierarchy, the young woman left behind her old social life and adopted the new order of the hospital. One nurse novel dramatized this moment. Walking down the hall with her class, a probationer catches sight of an old friend, an intern who had convinced her to enroll in the training school. When she greets him warmly, he rebuffs her, enforcing the hospital code of formality and distance.[34] As another new nurse discovers indignantly, the hospital's military respect for rank reversed the usual etiquette between men and women. "For the first time in my life, I'm stepping back from a door to let a man pass through first: Doctors first, always."[35]

The probationary period, usually about three to six months, tested the young woman's commitment to nursing and her fitness for the work. The transition from laywoman to nurse began in earnest when the neophyte first entered the ward. In the teens and early 1920s, student nurses often took on ward duties within their first week at the hospital, and some probationers were assigned to full twelve-hour shifts. Through the 1920s and 1930s, such long hours became less common, but students still spent at least two to four hours a day on the ward during their first months.[36] Set to work on menial tasks, the probationer underwent another form of ritual mortification and began to observe and adjust to hospital life.

One nurse, trained in the teens, humorously described her dawning awareness of a nurse's duties. "Who, I began to wonder, was to serve the lowly bedpans, hold the vomitus basins, change the smelly dressings, administer the blood transfusions and enemas?"[37] A nurse who entered school in 1912 recalled, "My first day was a trying one," an understated assessment of the nauseous task of cleaning up the operating room.[38] Another remembered her first day at school: she was sent to the operating room, where someone handed her an amputated foot to carry off.[39] Under such duress, young women quickly revised their romantic visions of holding patients' hands and soothing fevered brows.

The structure and content of probationers' work clearly indicated the schools' emphasis on practical over academic credentials. Before 1920, theoretical education was often provided by different physicians who lectured on their specialties in a loosely organized curriculum. Exhausted students could give only perfunctory attention to the lectures, which were held at night or during breaks in a twelve-hour shift. Students often seized the opportunity for some much-needed sleep. Most schools began to organize more systematic classroom work and to hire full-time nursing faculty in the 1920s and 1930s, but student nurses continued to provide most of the hospital nursing service through 1950.[40] Nursing arts—techniques of handling patients, giving routine care, and administering treatments—were taught in the classrooms, where students first practiced on "Mrs. Chase," the ubiquitous life-sized model, and then on each other. Later, on duty, students tested their skills under the supervision of an instructor or an advanced student, and gradually perfected their techniques in the constant repetition of the ward routine. Students had to perform credibly in their academic work, but the real test lay elsewhere.

Student nurses were evaluated after the first few months of probation, and the successful ones were honored in the ritual of capping. They still wore the stripes and pinafores of students, but they had attained the white caps that distinguished graduate nurses. They began to work full days on the ward, rotating through the hospital's different services. Soon after capping, the nurse took her first tour of night duty. Alone on the floor, she watched patients through the long hours of darkness. As a junior, or second-year, nurse, she might take charge of a busy ward during the day. Senior, or third-year, nurses, resplendent in their newly acquired whites, routinely ran the floors and helped to instruct less experienced students. At commencement, proud new nurses accepted their diplomas and the black bands that circle the white caps of graduate nurses.

To survive these rites of passage, the student had to acquire the stern discipline of the nurse. Strict rules of conduct offered young women a model of the controlled life. Her personal demeanor had to be schooled to the same standards. The impulsiveness of youth, the undisciplined license of lay life, had no place in the hospital. As the fictional Sue Barton begins her nursing career, a supervisor lectures the new students. "She has a grave responsibility and her manner should be in keeping with it. Personal adornment and personal pleasures must be put aside."[41] An ethics manual admonished, "The nurse must shun, while on duty, any suspicion of frivolity."[42] As another manual instructed, "It is all important, from the very outset, to study to keep well in hand one's various modes of expression and to watch them with unceasing diligence, until the habit of self-control becomes second nature."[43] Tempered by experience, this control would make the nurse equal to the challenges of hospital life.

Professional demeanor helped nurses to defend their emotions against the shocks of hospital life, and discipline guided their adjustment to unfamiliar and threatening situations. Both the physical intimacy of nursing and its psychological associations with sex and death made the work "dirty." Nurses' access to patients' bodies violated the boundaries of normal social relationships. They touched strangers and matter-of-factly dealt with their mucus, blood, urine, feces, vomitus, and bile. Nursing brought women into sustained contact with sickness and death, experiences that evoked fear and disgust in laypersons.[44] Through overt instruction and by example, student nurses learned inner discipline and shared rituals that helped to ward off their own uneasiness.

Memoirs and manuals contained anecdotes and special instructions on the hazards of male patients, acknowledging the cultural sensitivity of that relationship. As a long tradition of jokes, popular fiction, and pornography also shows, the nurse's physical contact with patients is charged with sexual associations. One ethics manual emphasizes the social anomaly of the young nurse's exposure to men's bodies: "Even men who have lived an evil life are troubled by such unusual circumstances."[45] Another nurse revealed the presence and threat of these sexual associations when asked if she had gotten any specific instructions about caring for male patients. A 1953 graduate, she laughed nervously and said, "Now how do you mean that? No, no, no, no, never, never, never—we were not *female*—we were *nurses*."[46]

Nurses were taught to use professional demeanor to dissociate themselves from the sexual intimations of physical contact. The nurse's professional poise and self-control framed the situation, marking it off from ordinary social encounters between men and women. Approaching her task impersonally, the young woman silently instructed her patient that their contact was strictly business. "No nurse can too soon learn the importance that tone and manner assume in such relations," one manual emphasized.[47] Others advised nurses to maintain their professional distance by avoiding "familiarity."[48] One admonished nurses never to tell patients their first names, and warned students that some patients might even "contrive to remove concealing drapes." Such advice defended the nurse's identity as a young woman from the contamination that patients might associate with her duties; as one discussion concluded, "Being a nurse in no way makes you less a lady."[49]

If male patients could fluster an inexperienced nurse, her exposure to sick and dying patients posed an even more severe trial to her self-control. In oral and written memoirs, nurses portray their early experiences with death in sharp detail. Often intense and deeply moving, sometimes grotesque or comical, these stories show how nurses learned to accept their responsibility for patients and to manage the emotional strain of death.

For many, hard work helped to control emotions that might otherwise have become overwhelming. Over and over, nurses explained that they overcame their fear of the responsibility of night duty by throwing themselves into their tasks. Confronted with emergencies, nurses discovered their resources for coping. One nurse who entered training in 1918 almost immediately faced overflowing wards and morgues as influenza struck her city. An inexperienced probationer, she learned quickly to lay out corpses: "It had to be done, so you did it."[50] Even under more ordinary circumstances, the busy routine of classes, ward duty, and study left little time for introspection.

More experienced nurses helped their charges to accept death as an inevitable part of their work. One nurse recalled the support of her supervising nurse during a difficult experience. As the hours crawled by on her first night duty, the student heard her patient lapse into Cheyne-Stokes respiration, the labored and erratic breathing of the dying. She called for the night supervisor, who questioned her about the patient's condition and then quietly confirmed the young woman's assessment. She asked the student about the nursing care she had given, and then concluded, "We have done everything we can to make this patient comfortable, but she is dying. There is nothing more you can do." In this understated way, the supervisor marked out the limits of nursing involvement. She commended the student for her careful observation and responsibility, and at the same time taught her to face a patient's impending death without guilt or panic.[51]

Supervisors tacitly acknowledged students' emotions in the face of death, but they insisted on self-control. One nurse's memoir described her lonely watch with a young dying patient and her overwhelming emotion as the end approached. She resolved, "I must steady myself. It will never do to go to pieces like this at the last moment." The child died soon after, and she carried his body to the morgue. Reporting the death to her night supervisor, she rebelled inwardly against the older woman's calmness, yet drew strength from her example. Later in the night, the supervisor stopped by to comfort the student, but gently told her that she must develop a nurse's self-command.[52] Another supervisor skillfully used the seniority system to bolster a quavering student. The young nurse controlled herself until her patient died, but then "became totally unstrung." She begged the head nurse not to leave her alone with the corpse, traditionally attended by a nurse until the undertaker arrived. The supervisor left the room but sent in "a little probationer. . . . Of course I tried to act brave then, for the sake of the other girl who had been there only a few days." Gradually she learned the nurse's stoic creed: "A nurse must take things as they come."[53]

Such counsel was not easy to live by. Nurses' narratives indicate the emotional strain of their work. Intriguingly, their memories of patients' deaths usually include physical descriptions that are vividly realistic, even naturalistic. Nurses frequently recalled the trauma of the nurse's last service to her patient, the physical care of the corpse. No doubt they remembered this experience because it was especially unfamiliar and shocking to them as students, and their frank accounts were a way for them to come to terms with death. By naming feared realities, nurses claimed control over them. Yet the content and tone of these narratives reveal a lingering uneasiness.

In memoirs, deathbed scenes often have supernatural intimations. Memorable deaths virtually always take place at night, with darkness and isolation creating an aura of mystery and suspense. Grotesque stories about unmanageable corpses dramatize nurses' confrontations with the physical reality of death. One early memoir recounts a senior nurse's frightful night on private duty outside the hospital. When her typhoid patient died, she prepared the body and settled down in a rocking chair to wait with it until morning. Suddenly she felt herself jerked backwards, jolted by the body, which had rolled off the bed onto the chair's rockers. "Even now I have a return of the horror of that moment," she wrote.[54] Others adopted gallows humor. A nurse trained in the 1940s drolly remembered struggling to move a large corpse with the inept assistance of a drunken orderly, who stumbled and tipped the stretcher over, dumping the heavy body on top of her.[55] Some stories have a nightmarish quality, portraying the nurse's struggle to free herself from the corpse and the painful emotions it evokes. A 1950s graduate remembered her complicated feelings of anger and sympathy for a male patient who died of lung cancer, and then recounted the unsettling experience of assisting at his autopsy. "I had to hold the airwick [a deodorizer] under the doctor's nose, I'll never forget that. They were supposed to cover his [the cadaver's] face, but [the drape] kept slipping off. . . . that was really hard to take, that was really awful."[56]

In their overtones of dread and guilt, these narratives reveal the price of self-control and the limits of reconciliation to death. The haunting images of dead patients dramatize the difficult, even contradictory, demands of professional demeanor. Self-control may be necessary, even exemplary, in the hospital, but in the world outside, equanimity in the face of suffering and death is somewhat suspect. The distance maintained by professional demeanor may protect nurses from overwhelming emotional involvement, but it also arouses discomfort and guilt. Physical care of the corpse powerfully evokes this charged issue, for when patients die, they become objects. One nurse's perceptive analysis, from a 1976 study of

nurses' responses to death, considers the meaning of her night-
mare of a deathbed scene: "What really hit me the first time I
took anyone to the morgue was that the stretcher they use
doesn't have any padding on it. You suddenly realize you're
no longer treating that person as a human being. What I heard
in the dream was sort of an angry response in a corpse coming
to life and chasing you because of what you're doing to them
or have done."[57] Vivid portrayals of uncooperative corpses
express nurses' guilt about their professional distance: in human outrage, the corpses refuse to behave as proper objects,
avenging themselves on the nurse. Such images are metaphors
for nurses' troubled responses to their patients' suffering and
their own needs for emotional distance.

Doctors and nurses both must learn to manage the
stresses of hospital life, and on the job, they develop the
common codes and comforts of sexual humor, ward camaraderie, and gallows humor. The bonds of shared work under
trying circumstances moderate and blur the lines of medical
hierarchy, for doctors and nurses alike are insiders, allied
against an uncomprehending laity. But although they have
much in common on the job, as men and women, doctors and
nurses bring different expectations and resources to the contradictory demands of professional demeanor. Narratives of
medical apprenticeship, like nurses' stories, show young doctors confronting the unsettling realities of hospital life. But
male doctors frequently respond by cultivating a stance of
cynicism and bravado, an option forged from cultural prescriptions for unflinching manhood.[58] Whatever the emotional
costs of such a choice, it does not set work and gender roles at
odds. Doctors, like professionals generally, are men writ
large: decisive, stoical, objective. As women, nurses have to
defy the conventions of gender to meet the demands of hospital discipline, renouncing cultural prescriptions for female
warmth and emotional expressiveness. Pulled between the
demands of work and the cultural construction of gender,
nurses express considerable ambivalence about the prescribed
objectivity.

Manuals, novels, and prescriptive literature indicate the tension between prescriptions for work and for gender; to a striking degree, they dwell on the troublesome issue of professional demeanor. The ideology of discipline countered and challenged the dominant culture by inculcating young women with an image of female strength. Narratives of initiation during hospital apprenticeship show students overcoming the conflict between work and gender in resolutions that affirm women's control and competence on the job.

The literature struggled with the problem of maintaining professional demeanor and warned of the pitfalls of callousness and sentimentality, two words that constantly recur. Manuals tacitly acknowledged cultural claims on women in advising young nurses to guard against becoming hardened and cynical.[59] Similarly, the authors of nursing novels addressed the cultural anomaly of female detachment through characters who were novices. In the novel *Into the Wind*, for example, a new student observes her more seasoned roommates with mixed feelings. "They're as human as your own family when they're grousing about having to get out of bed, and they're as—as impersonal as lamp-posts when they're ready to go *on*, as they call it."[60] In the same fashion, the spirited probationer of a fictionalized memoir reflects doubtfully on the advice to remain objective: "I was deeply moved as I looked into her patient little face, wondering how a nurse could reconcile her two separate selves, one the indifferent, cold, calculating creature who took things impersonally, held fast to rules, crowded out all impulses of kindness: and the other gentle, tolerant, patient, and understanding."[61]

Prescriptive literature sometimes counseled the student to seek the serenity of religion as her ballast and guide. One manual advised, "The nearer to her heart she keeps the teachings and the life of Christ in her everyday work, the greater will be her strength to overcome difficulties and to forget herself in helping others."[62] In a 1946 didactic novel written by a nurse, a fatherly doctor listens to a young nurse recite her professional ideals and piously reminds her, " 'Pity,

helpfulness, understanding . . . . Those are Christian virtues
. . . they will wither and die unless they are fed from Christian
sources."[63] But most of the prescriptive literature tacitly acknowledged the failing power of such ideology. In some
manuals, advice about the nurse's spiritual life was vague and
perfunctory, while the authors of others addressed their secular audiences in resigned or defensive tones. One reminded her
readers not to forget "the old-fashioned habit of going to
church,"[64] and another noted, "In hospital work there is a
tendency to forget that we are not entirely physical beings."[65]
A 1936 manual admonished students, "No girl is so all-
sufficient that she needs no contact with the Unseen," yet
revealed the minority status of even such an ecumenical deity
with its concluding advice: "Do not be ashamed to have your
associates know that you still have faith in spiritual values."[66]
While schools with religious affiliations undoubtedly gave the
Lord His due in more confident affirmations, religion occupied an increasingly marginal position in most of the nursing
literature.

In place of religious faith was a pragmatic ideology that
directed nurses to earthly goals, motivating them to learn
emotional control for the sake of success in work. Prescriptive
literature resisted the negative connotations of professional
demeanor for women, rejecting the layperson's association of
self-control with callousness. Didactic stories and advice left
no room for doubt: the nurse had to achieve emotional discipline to do her work. This message appeared so predictably in
manuals, memoirs, and novels that it sometimes took on a
rehearsed quality, as one nurse's recollections illustrate: "We
soon learned that we could not be nurses of calm judgment and
steady nerves unless we detached ourselves entirely from the
personal element in every case," she explained. "This does not
mean that we were callous to human suffering but rather that
we sought to relieve our feelings by skillful help rather than
through emotion."[67] Such control carried personal costs, as
these sources conceded implicitly, but the rewards and satisfactions of successful nursing would outweigh the losses.

Initiation narratives powerfully reinforced this ideology. They portrayed students who resolve their doubt and ambivalence about professional distance in the certainty of a full commitment to nursing. In *Into the Wind*, for example, student nurse Sabra first learns the rules of professional objectivity in the classroom. Back in her room, she wonders aloud how to reconcile this unaccustomed detachment with her own images of womanly compassion. Her roommate irreverently advises, "All I can say is get disillusioned as quickly as possible and save yourself whatever you can in the process. It can be pretty ghastly." Other experienced students chime in to corroborate bluntly, shocking Sabra with their complaints and cynicism about ward duty. But underneath these rough exteriors, her seniors show the spirit of professional commitment. "It's worth it all the day you get your cap," they assure her. "Then you know you're part of something that has purpose."[68]

Bitter experience teaches Sabra the pitfalls of her sentimental attitude. Despite the warnings she receives, Sabra grows intensely involved with a patient whose illness mystifies the doctors. Upset about the patient's suffering, she becomes distracted and clumsy on the ward. She retreats to the utilities' room for a probationer's moment of truth: "I've wasted this whole three months. I haven't learned the most rudimentary thing about nursing, for I haven't learned to keep my head. I haven't learned not to let things get on a personal level . . . . and that's the very thing Miss Wilbur has warned us about time and again. She told us it would ball up our work, and it certainly does."[69] As she learns to control her emotions, she reasons through the patient's case and, in a triumphant conclusion, helps to make the diagnosis.

Similarly, *I Was a Probationer* traces a student's exposure to professional demeanor and her gradual acceptance of its underlying ideology. An intern observes the young nurse's dismay at a child's death and tells her, "You'll be able to take it as part of your work in time . . . . Time makes all of us callous . . . . If we let our emotions carry us away, we might not be able to do for the patient what must be done." As she learns to care for a badly burned patient, her senior nurse warns her about the excruciating pain she will inflict when she changes the dressings, and advises, "Now don't go under. Just remember it's another case. Say to yourself that you are trying to relieve suffering, that everything is being done that is humanly possible. I know how you'll feel."[70]

As her training progresses, the student acquires the discipline of hospital life, and affirms the value of control. Nursing a patient with advanced gangrene, she reflects, "Two months before, I would have been revolted at the sight of her rotting foot, but now I accepted it without letting it touch me emotionally. That was the way nurses became callous to suffering, and I was beginning to see that it was a fortunate adjustment. Otherwise they could not endure the demands made upon them." This initiation is complete when she and her classmate begin to pass on the lesson to the new entering class. When a naive probationer gives an emotionally colored account of her patient's plight, the seasoned students admonish her sharply. "It's all right to have a certain amount of pity for suffering, but there's nothing about a pan of saffron vomit that makes me feel sentimental. Forget your feelings. You've got to face the repulsive side as well as the sentimental."[71]

Didactic fiction often dramatized the culmination of apprenticeship, the moment when a student comes to identify herself as a nurse. Confronted with the test of a sudden emergency, Sue Barton thinks quickly and saves the day. She takes pride in this evidence of her developing skill and competence, and stops to reflect on her gradual transformation from laywoman to nurse when she returns briefly to her old world. On a short visit home, she feels distant from her once-familiar circle of family and friends. "Her real life was in the hospital now . . . . Invisible cords bound her to it, for she was a born nurse. She knew it, now."[72] Some accounts explicitly pose the conflict between work and private life, especially romance. In one fictional example, Cherry Ames, the heroine of a series of nursing adventures, is called from the Christmas dance to cover a short-staffed floor. Changing from her black lace dress to hospital whites, she feels inspired by a new sense of duty. "The hospital uniform came first."[73] The story "The Birth of a Nurse" captured the same moment. The protagonist, a junior nurse, is called to assist at an emergency just as she and her friend are leaving the hospital for a party. At first disappointed, she becomes deeply involved in the case. When her friend returns to console her for missing the fun, the nurse finds herself feeling a bit superior to her companion, who suddenly seems childish. "How could she explain to Eleanor this feeling she never had before? This knowledge of what really mattered . . . . 'To think I helped!' "[74] Nursing commitment meant initiation into adulthood. In "A Cadet Gets Her Cap," a young nurse thinks soberly, "I wasn't the same girl I had been five months ago. Almost I wasn't a girl at all. I was a woman, a nurse and I had been given a charge to keep."[75] Such stories ran against cultural prescriptions for women, and indeed against a broader cultural emphasis on private life and leisure, to affirm the value of satisfying work.

One common feature of student culture suggests another level at which young women sought to resolve the conflicts between gender and work. Leaving their old identities behind, students frequently coined new names for one another. Memoirs and novels provide many examples. An especially rich source is the column "Calling All Nurses," a regular feature in RN that printed letters from nurses trying to locate former classmates or co-workers. In virtually every example, these names were neuter or masculine, perhaps symbolizing students' recognition of the "masculine" character of their work. Nurses often addressed their peers by their last names. Very likely this usage developed as an irreverent abbreviation of the hospital etiquette, which mandated formality. Common among men, the familiar use of last names was more unusual for women. Nurses also dubbed each other with inventive nicknames. Female or feminine tags were very rare; one "Mother" Mount stood out from dozens of others. Sometimes pet names came from the medical language nurses shared; one pair of students named themselves "Morphine" and "Atropine." Many others were masculine diminutives, usually invented from students' surnames: Gertrude Peterson answered to "Pete," Iona McCoy was called "Mac," Helen L. Donoghue was "Donnie," and "Althea" was quickly shortened to "Al." Others resolutely defied gender classification, like "Smoky" Phillips, "Wicky" (Olive Wagner), and "Mergie" (Elsie M. Bernhoft). In renaming one another, student nurses selected names that pushed feminine associations into the background.[76]

This distinctive culture did not go unchallenged as the enclosed female world of the hospital school became increasingly anachronistic. More colleges and universities began admitting "co-eds," the developing field of psychology celebrated romantic heterosexuality, and popular culture and social life focused more and more on the heterosexual couple.[77] Responding uneasily to the mounting pressure on same-sex institutions, manuals advised students to moderate their relationships with other women. Overt references to homosexuality appear even in early prescriptive literature—even though nursing courses did not include basic material on sex and birth control until the 1950s and 1960s.

A 1900 manual cautioned, "Towards fellow probationers and the other nurses in the ward it is best not to be too familiar or too friendly; sudden, violent friendships are undesirable and unnecessary. . . . Sentimental, intense personal friendships between nurses are a mistake. . . . In some instances they must be regarded as forms of perverted affection; they are always unhealthy, since they make too great demands upon the emotions and nerve force, and are likely to assume undue proportions."[78] A 1936 manual counseled, "Do not pick out one or two girls as special friends, but make friends of them all. Under no circumstances permit yourself to have a 'crush' upon another girl. It does not look well, it will be misinterpreted, and it may cause jealousy."[79] *Emotional Hygiene*, written in the late 1940s, urged student nurses to avoid the wayside of homosexuality in "the procession headed toward emotional maturity." "Do not let anyone who is biologically arrested there, hinder you from making your own progress. Some who have been unwittingly drawn into homosexual acts have thereafter . . . felt unworthy of normal adult love."[80] Such warnings were the most extreme expressions of the conflict between gender and work: the commitment to work was so anomalous for women that it might threaten heterosexuality itself.

Nonetheless, in a culture that defined love and marriage as the center of women's lives, the hospital schools, prescriptive literature, and nurses all affirmed the choice of work over marriage. One nurse remembered her decision to enter training school thus: "I was feeling serious—like a nun about to take the veil."[81] Ethics manuals extolled the solid satisfactions of professional life, and urged students to approach their work "as single-mindedly as if there were no question that their lives were to be given to professional activities. The possibility of matrimony has wrecked many a career by hovering about the young woman, distracting her interest and proving in the end to be an illusion."[82] Didactic novels explicitly carried this advice into the years after graduation. For nurses in fiction, the inducements of marriage paled before the excitement of work and the company of other nurses. After graduation, Cherry Ames and her classmates enlist in the army, and then take an apartment together in New York, where they gather for reunions throughout the dozens of novels in the series. Eternally single, Cherry adroitly evades her many boyfriends once their thoughts turn to matrimony. Sue Barton refuses to marry her ardent suitor, a dedicated young doctor, so she can spend a year nursing with Kit, her close friend and former classmate. As they move into their new apartment, Sue complains about a missing classmate. "I wish Connie were here. . . . Darn it—why does she have to get married so soon—just when we're beginning to do things."[83] Sue's own marriage later takes her away from Kit for a year, but then she and her husband persuade Kit to become the superintendent of nurses at his rural hospital. By the next book, Sue is back at work, this time as a staff nurse in her friend's nursing service.

The ideology and experience of training school reverberated in women's lives and work. Many nurses apparently shared the strong identification with their work that fiction and memoirs describe. As one nurse wrote in 1941, "There's something about nursing that gets into the blood."[84] A married nurse who decided to return to work corroborated, "Giving up nursing is much harder than it might seem . . . this profession gets a 'hold' on you."[85] For these nurses, apprenticeship culture nurtured the intense commitment to work that is more commonly associated with professional training and practice. In oral memoirs, even women who had not been employed for many years continued to identify themselves and to be identified by others as nurses. Frequently, neighbors and family drew on their skills and experiences, asking nurses about child-raising problems or illness in the family and summoning them in emergencies. Some nurses used their skills in community agencies. One woman worked as a volunteer for the local visiting nurses' association, and a day care center solicited her for its board because she was a nurse.[86] And most talked wistfully of going back to work someday. Nursing remained a part of them in a way that other women's work simply does not: waitresses, secretaries, teachers, or social workers seldom have such strong and enduring personal and social connections to their work. Memoirs and letters often corroborate the messages of prescriptive literature and fiction; as one editorial put it, "No true nurse ever really stops nursing though she may be far afield in her daily work. In her heart she is always a nurse."[87]

Implicitly and overtly, the literature and culture of apprenticeship subverted the dominant ideology of woman's place. First, narratives of initiation undercut cultural ideals by testing prescribed characteristics of "femininity" against the demands of hospital life. As young women converted to the nursing creed, they came to see delicacy and refinement as mere squeamishness, and to view emotional expressiveness as suspect, often a sign of weak and facile sentimentality. Hospital discipline replaced these superficial responses with the mature realism of the nurse. Second, in a culture that valued women primarily in domestic roles, the schools presented the attractions of work outside the home. In their positive portrayals of women's competence, seriousness, and emotional control, the narratives promoted female commitment to work.

In the self-contained world of the hospital schools, such values could flourish. Set apart from the social life of their contemporaries, young women participated in a communal life arranged around work. Theirs was a woman's world: they enjoyed the support and camaraderie of other women as peers, and looked up to female models as they worked with more experienced students and supervisors. Few other institutions in the twentieth century could provide young women with a comparable experience of female autonomy. Seldom explicitly feminist in their ideology, the schools nonetheless empowered young nurses as women by expecting much of them, and by denying the cultural contradiction between femininity and commitment to work.

III. COLLEGE DEGREES: THE HAVES AND THE HAVE-NOTS

Until World War II, superintendents and graduates of the diploma schools coexisted with nursing leaders or self-styled nurse-educators, who sought university training for nurses. Occasional clashes indicated the sensitivity of the issue, but the movement toward degrees was too slight to threaten the hospital schools or their defenders. With the war, leaders gained a new advantage. Wartime needs for mobilization and central coordination brought the professional associations a new national visibility and prominence. Rank-and-file nurses watched anxiously as small committees quietly began to plan for two-tiered nursing education after the war. Concerned with leaders' growing emphasis on degrees for nurses in teaching and supervisory positions, the editor of *Trained Nurse* asked, "Do we mean that we want to create two classes of

RNs—bedside nurses and officers?"[88] A letter from "Retired Nurse" put the case even more bluntly. "Those with degrees get the bossing jobs. Those without degrees roll up their sleeves. I think there is a distinct class consciousness between the haves and the have-nots. Is this what we want? Do we mean that every nurse should have a degree? If so, why not say so right out loud?"[89]

When leaders did endorse this policy after the war, adopting the 1948 Brown report as their manifesto, hospital superintendents and diploma graduates became increasingly uneasy. In a letter headed "Will Nurses without College Degrees Be Wanted?" a nurse who signed herself simply "RN, New York" confided, "I have a great feeling of insecurity. . . . I am unhappy and know that others in similar positions are asking, 'What does the future hold for me?'"[90] Stung by leaders' dismissal of the apprenticeship tradition, many nurses lashed out against the new proposals. Protesting nurses defended the craft skills of nursing arts, hurt and angry at their demotion to "technical" nurses. "It's not the university graduate who knows how to give a better back rub or how to administer to the patient's comfort in countless ways, but the nurse who has been trained for it and who does not feel too far superior to carry out the everyday tasks."[91] Another nurse weighed "Inherent Nursing Values vs. Professional Snobbery," concluding that patient care was deteriorating as nursing education moved from the bedside.[92] In this recurring theme, nurses defended the value and complexity of good bedside care, resisting leaders' view of the "professional" nurse as manager, responsible for patient care but not at the bedside herself. Such nurses criticized leaders for forsaking nurses' traditional skills and identity in a vain effort to imitate the status and prerogatives of physicians. "Too much theory and too little practice of nursing procedures may produce a pseudo-doctor who will be neither an aid nor a comfort to the sick patient," warned one nurse, who had a degree but hastened to dissociate herself from the Brown report.[93] Another concluded that "we have become entirely too college wacky. . . . We need . . . more and better nurses to care for the patient—and fewer doctorettes."[94]

Rank-and-file nurses also protested the elitism of the professional associations, criticizing the ANA both for its internal operation and the educational program it endorsed. Many nurses felt disenfranchised by the rapid move toward college education. The recommendations of the Brown report were never voted upon by the ANA or NLNE membership, and indeed never formally adopted by either organization, yet the report became the basis for a new classification and accreditation program. Critics of college education censured leaders for this arbitrary action, which one author labeled "authoritarianism in nursing." Other observers charged that the new standards would discourage many prospective or practicing nurses at a time of shortage. If leaders succeeded, young women could no longer enter nursing unless they had the money for college tuition, and experienced nurses would have to leave their jobs and rearrange family responsibilities to earn degrees.[95]

In their support for apprenticeship, superintendents and graduates defended their own histories and their jobs against an upgrading that threatened to leave them behind. They confronted leaders' strivings for credentials with a stubborn craft pride, valuing their work for what it was instead of yearning for what it might become. Over the next years, their fears about the future would be painfully confirmed. Rising standards would make it harder for young women to become nurses, R.N.s without degrees would face constricting opportunities for jobs and promotions, the nursing hierarchy would grow more elaborate and rigid, the division of labor in hospitals would disrupt the traditional craft of nursing arts.

Yet in the end, apprenticeship itself could not be defended. Nurses needed more theoretical training to meet the new demands of their work and to defend themselves as workers in a changing context. As patient care became more complex, partially trained student nurses were increasingly inadequate to carry primary responsibility for the nursing service. Advances of World War II spurred the growth of medical technology and science, and therapeutics changed rapidly as new knowledge suggested new approaches to treatment. In a situation where specific technical skills might become rapidly outmoded, nurses simply had to have the tools of theoretical thinking. The hospital schools had moved a long way in this direction by 1950, but the structure of apprenticeship set inexorable limits on the expansion of nurses' academic education. The schools were subject to administrators' financial analyses, for hospitals could not maintain schools indefinitely unless they could accrue some benefit to themselves. To justify operating schools, hospital administrators had to use students as workers. Although the schools had more coherent curriculums by the 1950s, academic education still got short shrift as class and study time competed with hours on duty.

Nursing education also had to change to keep up with women's changing work patterns. In the 1920s, most working nurses were young and single. About half were under thirty years old, and a generous estimate suggested that only one in five active nurses was married. Although some nurses remained at work for many years, over half of all graduates left nursing after ten years.[96] By 1950, nurses were staying at work longer, and the average working woman was older. Married nurses constituted 42 percent of active nurses, and less than 40 percent were under thirty.[97] In the early years, nursing care stayed up to date largely by infusions of new workers, trained in recent methods and techniques. But as individual nurses stayed at work longer and encountered rapid changes in care, they needed the flexibility of broader training.

Nor could apprenticeship training withstand the diverse pressures of postwar social life; nursing had to adjust to the new choices and constraints of women's lives. Nurses' training had once offered one of the few post-high school educational courses available to women. By 1950, more women could consider college; thus, to continue recruiting the upwardly mobile working-class woman or the middle-class woman, nursing schools had to compete with college and university courses. Broader social changes also undercut the whole style and character of the hospital schools. The austere life of the hospital had grown increasingly anachronistic since the turn of the century. The rise of fascism before the war, and the expansion of the Soviet bloc after the war, made Americans fearful of both the left and the right, and they reacted with suspicion toward anything resembling regimentation. During the virulent anticommunism of the 1950s, critics began to react against the strict discipline of nursing schools, charging hospitals with "authoritarianism." In any case, discipline had little appeal to young women exposed to the enticements of leisure and consumer culture; increasingly the strictures of nursing school were unfavorably compared to the light-hearted years of the college co-ed. And, sadly, as the feminine mystique took hold, the schools' emphasis on commitment to work came under attack with heightened demands for education to prepare women for life as wives and mothers.[98]

Superintendents and graduates had little chance of diverting the tide that pressed nursing toward college education. While they recognized and criticized the elitism of leaders' programs, they never developed a coherent alternative to meet the challenges of their changing technological and social context. Without a women's movement and the explicitly feminist ideology it could have provided, they could not articulate and claim the schools' legacy in supporting women's autonomy. Instead, many became entangled in reacting against nursing's leadership. In the end, these nurses ironically found themselves aligned with the more conservative doctors and hospital managers, "allies" who often supported hospital schools for reasons that ultimately undermined the interests of nurses.

The National Organization of Hospital Schools of Nursing (NOHSN) was a case in point. Founded in October 1949, the organization sought to stop the momentum of the Brown report by preserving apprenticeship education. The group challenged the new national accrediting system, asserted its support for all hospital schools that met existing minimum standards of state boards, and vowed to defend the diploma programs in their "struggle for survival." It also opposed federal funding for nurses' training in defense of local autonomy and private medicine. In a leap familiar to the conservative American Medical Association, the NOHSN linked the success of these causes to the survival of the free world. It successfully lobbied against the Emergency Professional Health Training Act of 1949, legislation that would have provided money for nurses' education.[99]

Other opponents of the Brown recommendations frequently dismissed college education in terms that slighted nurses as workers and as women. Outspoken doctors and administrators denounced leaders for restricting access to training during the postwar shortage, but along with their concern for the public good they also revealed their frank disregard for nurses' special skills. The American Surgical Association countered the Brown report by proposing a shorter two-year course for nurses, flatly asserting, "Years of higher education are not required to supply [nursing care], despite the unwise aims of national nursing bodies."[100] The American Hospital Association's retiring president, Graham L. Davis, made a blistering speech at the 1948 AHA convention, attacking the Brown recommendations in rhetoric that displayed his own views of nurses and of women. Reviving the time-honored special-fitness argument, he urged that all girls should learn nursing arts from childhood on. After high school graduation, they could take a few months' apprenticeship in hospitals to complete their training. Thus prepared, they could make themselves useful until marriage removed them to higher duties.[101]

Platitudes about public service and womanly duty joined conveniently with more concrete administrative interests. Many hospital managers were loath to give up the social control they had enjoyed with the apprenticeship system.

They did not represent a clear majority; managerial strategies were changing in the 1940s and 1950s, as administrators began to question the purpose and utility of maintaining schools (see Chapter 5). Still, many remained outspoken defenders of student staffs, and their motives were not necessarily narrowly economic. One administrator claimed that his school ran at a deficit, but he maintained it as a valuable asset in "building morale." Students' esprit de corps helped to inspire other workers to identify with the hospital family, and "as everyone knows, loyalty is one quality in an employee that cannot be bought with money."[102]

Some feared that education outside the hospital, especially college education, might encourage young women to reach above themselves and to make troublesome demands at work. In confronting this threat, managers could appeal to the postwar concern for "stability" to legitimate a conservative ethos. Similarly, the new interest in narrowly vocational education could be enlisted in the service of maintaining the status quo. The Ginzberg report, a sociological study of nursing published in 1948, reflected the postwar philosophy of "life-adjustment" education and showed its conservative implications:

> It is not sound educational and personnel practice to train people to a degree beyond the opportunities they will have to utilize their training effectively in their work. Nursing cannot offer sufficient opportunities for all its members to make fairly constant use of advanced knowledge and specialized skills. The war proved on a large scale what private industry had long known on a much smaller scale—that a more serious source of discontent among employees is a conspicuous under-utilization of their talent and skills.[103]

While leaders sought to expand nurses' opportunities, such arguments aimed to shape the worker to fit the limited possibilities of work as it was.

Similarly, some doctors defended diploma programs because they feared that the college-educated nurse would threaten their authority. One doctor complained that the collegiate programs placed too much emphasis on assessment and judgment, therefore infringing on the physician's prerogative of diagnosis. He reminded nurses that "the doctor is the coach of the team—and to a large extent the quarter-back also."[104] Medical associations took the ball and ran with it. While the American Medical Association did not take a formal stance against the Brown report, the organization consistently opposed nursing leaders' efforts to close diploma schools. Individual doctors and state and local medical groups raised nurses' ire with criticisms of college education.

Differences over funding divided doctors and nursing leaders even more sharply. Viewing any state involvement as a threat to private medicine, the AMA opposed aid for nurses' education. Physicians defended their own fee-for-service arrangements and private practice at a time when more and more nurses were leaving private duty for salaried positions. Though some nurses supported doctors in their resistance to "socialized medicine," others began to defect quietly. The World War II Cadet Nurse Corps program indicated the advantages of outside funding for nurses, and leaders worked to claim more federal money after the war. The AMA opposed the ANA's bid for federal funding, and unfailingly lobbied against bills that brought federal money into nursing programs.[105]

By making the argument about nursing education strictly utilitarian, administrators and doctors denied leaders' claims for upward mobility, for expanded authority on the job, for more recognition of the value of women's work. College education in America has never been purely vocational; it represents also both a vehicle for upward mobility and, however imperfectly and partially, a tradition of humanistic values, of learning for its own sake. To argue that nurses did not "need" college education was to confirm their secondary status as workers and as women.

Along with their conservative allies, dissenting nurses largely neglected the feminist dimensions of the issue. Hospital school graduates took pride in their diplomas, yet many also wished later that they had had more academic education. Two nurses chorused, "I can't imagine doing any other kind of work," but one added wistfully that she regretted not having a "more rounded training," and the other made up her mind to get it, enrolling in a college program twenty-five years after her graduation from nursing school.[106] College education could open a new and wider world for women. "E.E.," a public-health nurse, wrote *AJN* to praise postgraduate education. She had returned reluctantly to school when told she needed more theoretical work, and found herself enthralled "to learn the joy of 'just knowing.'"[107] Another nurse warmly remembered her work at Teachers College, a stimulating change from her quiet rural girlhood and the protected years of training school. "[It was] the most exciting experience in the whole world. . . . They really wanted nurses to have more, and to know about more, than just nursing."[108] In their bitterness over the Brown report, nurses sometimes overlooked the opportunities that college could provide. Correctly identifying the degree as a restrictive credential, they chose to fight against collegiate education rather than to struggle to make it more accessible.

Leaders, too, failed to defend women's claims to education when they tried to make the degree an entry-level credential without building bridges to it for diploma nurses. Some of the difficulties of the transition were perhaps inevitable, but much of diploma nurses' insecurity and anger could have been averted with a more generous and inclusive program of upgrading. Instead, leaders calculated on the basis of nurses' high attrition; in ten or twenty years, most non-degree nurses would no longer be practicing, and nursing's ranks could be filled with a new breed of college-educated young women. Meanwhile, those nurses who wished to advance at work had to sacrifice their own time and income for degrees. Leaders were slow to explore and support arrangements that would help diploma nurses to earn degrees, options such as programs of in-service education, contract demands for educational benefits, or advanced placement based on nursing school courses and work experience. Because there were few available routes for upgrading, the new requirements sometimes imposed real hardships on nurses already at work. College became a sorting mechanism that devalued hard-won skills and blocked diploma nurses' upward mobility.

Embroiled in conflict over professionalization, both leaders and their opponents lost sight of the larger meaning of women's education. Both could have learned from the counsel of Lavinia Dock, an early nursing leader, suffragist, and feminist, who wrote in 1909: "The thing of real importance is not that nurses should be taught less, but that all women should be taught more."[109] The "haves" and the "have-nots" could also have learned from one another. Defending apprenticeship education, supporters of the hospital schools failed to seize on the opportunities of a changing situation in which college education was becoming more widely available than ever before. Leaders understood and responded to postwar possibilities, but they were all too ready to abandon the majority of nurses in pursuit of professionalization. As a result, education became a deeply divisive issue that virtually split nurses into two occupational cultures. Guided by professional ideology, leaders had little sympathy or understanding for the values and codes of apprenticeship. Yet on the job, most nurses would derive their sense of nursing's meaning and purpose from the culture of apprenticeship, not from the premises of professional ideology. Confronting their common problems as women and as workers, nurses would often find themselves speaking different languages.

CHAPTER 3

The Freelance Nurse: Private Duty from 1920 to World War II

In the 1920s and 1930s, most nurses graduated from the bustling wards of hospital training schools to work in private duty, caring for a single patient at home or in the hospital. Unlike salaried public-health or hospital nurses, private-duty nurses operated as freelancers: their patients hired them and paid them by the shift or by the day. Nurses found their cases through hospital or private registries, which acted as employment bureaus. Doctors, nursing superintendents, and patients applied to the registries, which matched these requests with their lists of nurses on call. Informal and often highly personal, the hiring networks and job situation of private duty nursing preserved much of the atmosphere of nineteenth-century domestic nursing.

The powerful, central position of hospitals in medical care today has all but obscured this history. The word "nursing" evokes images of white-clad women in antiseptic hospital settings, but until World War II, private duty was the core of nursing work. Few graduate nurses were hired to work on hospital staffs, and jobs in hospital administration and public health were largely restricted to nurses with more education or with diplomas from elite nursing schools. In 1920, 70 to 80 percent of all nurses worked in private duty. Such work amounted almost to another common experience of initiation, for even nurses who ended up in hospital or public-health jobs usually began their careers in private duty. Freelance nurses served a broad public. Memoirs and surveys indicate that private duty was not exclusively or even primarily the privilege of the wealthy. Before 1930, many accounts portray the freelance nurse in a variety of workplaces, from lavish homes to crowded tenements and broken-down rural shacks. While the poorest families would call a nurse only *in extremis*, private-duty nursing was a commonplace accompaniment to illness in middle- and upper-class households. Such patients routinely called private nurses to attend minor ailments, convalescence, and childbirth, as well as when more serious illness struck. Private duty, then, played a prominent role in nursing as an occupation and in the layperson's experience of health care.[1]

The changing context and experience of private-duty nursing in the 1920s and 1930s illuminate nurses' transition to the hospital workplace and the gradual eclipse of freelance practice. The years just before and after World War I created an aura of promise around private-duty nursing, a sense of expanding horizons that accurately indicated the new legitimacy of the trained nurse and her work, but that proved illusory for the specific form of freelance practice. As the United States moved toward war with Germany, a national call for mobilization of nurses brought a sense of urgency and importance to the hospital schools, and the rapid production of new nurses continued unabated. In the influenza pandemic of 1918–19, lay and medical authorities urged young women to enter nursing. After the armistice, growing medical and lay demands for private nursing services seemed to promise a solid peacetime market to absorb the still-growing numbers of trained nurses. When the enrollment of student nurses dropped after the war, memories of the epidemic and of wartime scarcities brought alarmed cries of a nursing shortage. But the transitional years between the wars brought new developments in medical care and hospital organization that undercut private-duty nursing, even as broader social and economic shifts began to narrow its clientele. Although the majority of nurses worked as freelancers until World War II, such nurses were increasingly relegated to the margins of the emerging system of specialized care centered in hospitals. During World War II, the hospital asserted its dominance over nursing practice in decisive terms: since the 1940s, hospitals have claimed more nurses than any other employer. For the graduate of the 1920s, nursing meant private duty; for her counterpart of the 1940s, it meant work on a hospital ward. The transition from private duty to hospital staff work poised nursing between the claims of an older craft organization and the newer imperatives of rationalization. Even under the adverse conditions of the 1920s and 1930s, private-duty nurses struggled to maintain their prerogatives as freelance workers. Acutely aware of the growing constraints on private-duty nursing, they still resisted employment in hospitals. In defending the organization of private duty as it was, they ran up against leaders' efforts to place nurses in salaried hospital jobs. Once again, leaders astutely assessed nursing's position in a changing situation: by the 1920s, private duty *was* obsolete, a relic of more personal and informal arrangements for health care in a system that had yielded to medical professionalization and hospital growth. But again, in failing to address the immediate needs of most nurses, leaders pursued long-term goals alone and against the weight of their colleagues' opposition. And just as they had overlooked the contributions of apprenticeship training, they were prone to slight the private-duty nurse's preference of more individual nursing care and her fierce defense of nurses' autonomy at work.

I. THE PERILS OF PRIVATE DUTY

The work lives of private-duty nurses before 1930 illustrate both the advantages and the insecurities of their freelance status. Arrangements for hiring nurses were often highly informal, and, under favorable circumstances, individual nurses could exert considerable control over the pace and timing of their work. But being isolated and unorganized, private-duty nurses also proved acutely vulnerable to fluctuations in the market. When employment conditions worsened, their fragile independence collapsed. Facing the rapid obsolescence of their

services and largely unsupported by professional leaders, private-duty nurses could not hope to regain their old positions.

On the face of it, the arrangements of private duty resembled the celebrated independence of craft workers.[2] As freelance workers, nurses could schedule cases to suit their own
needs and preferences. They could take time off to rest after a
tiring stint, or take themselves off the registrar's list temporar-
ily if sick friends or relatives needed their help. Freelance
arrangements also gave nurses the opportunity to evade unappealing work situations, a prerogative they exercised freely.
Private-duty nurses constantly thwarted the registrars' efforts
to impose discipline and order by picking and choosing
among cases the registrar offered. Doctors, nursing leaders,
and registrars complained bitterly about that practice. One
survey indicated that 61 percent of nurses routinely refused
certain types of cases, baldly listing their restrictions with the
registrar. Contagious, obstetrical, and mental cases were the
most unpopular; smaller numbers of nurses refused night
cases, twenty-four–hour duties, home cases, or male patients.
Undoubtedly even more "case-picking" occurred on an informal basis, for a nurse could declare herself off duty if confronted with an unappealing prospect.[3]

Less often, private-duty nurses could manage their relationships with doctors and patients so as to enhance their
control at work. Some nurses formed informal partnerships
with friendly doctors, and enjoyed the security of a steady
clientele and a congenial working relationship. Nurses could
also avoid doctors whom they found troublesome. One nurse
reported indignantly that an independent colleague of hers had
registered against seven different doctors, "because *she* does
not approve of their methods."[4] A well-established nurse
enjoyed a special status in her community, and could set her
own terms with patients who found "their" nurse an indispensable aid in illness or childbirth. One highly regarded
private-duty nurse, for example, was in such demand that her
obstetrical patients had to make appointments for their next
baby's projected arrival while the nurse attended the current

convalescence. If they did not produce the next offspring on schedule and failed to cancel their reservation, the nurse charged them for her time.[5]

On the job, private duty gave nurses considerable autonomy in their work habits. In principle, of course, the same rules of discipline governed all nurses. In home cases, the nurse was subject to the authority of the patient's doctor; in hospitals, private-duty nurses fell under the purview of the superintendent, who was formally responsible for all nursing care in her institution. But in practice, private-duty nurses worked with little supervision. Doctors visited their home patients, but did not stay to oversee the nurse. Hospital nursing services sometimes had rules about the "special nurses" who cared for private patients; for example, a hospital might specify the amount of relief time that a private-duty nurse could expect from students or graduates working on the same floor. But in the actual work situation, busy head nurses rarely interfered with the bedside care that special nurses provided. Outside the rigid hierarchy of the hospital, they escaped the discipline and demands of institutional work. No time-and-motion experts dogged their footsteps; no clumsy interns or demanding doctors disrupted their nursing routines. As one nurse declared with satisfaction, "I am my own boss."[6]

But the exercise of this autonomy was a highly individualistic and somewhat uncertain affair under the best of circumstances. A closer look reveals the narrow economic and social margin within which the freelance nurse's independence could flourish. To support themselves as freelance workers, private-duty nurses had to establish a steady clientele. Dependent on hospitals, registries, and community ties for their referrals, nurses had to contend with the intense loyalties of alumnae networks and cater to the demands of local doctors and patients. Hospital registries favored alumnae of their own schools, placing "outside" nurses at the bottom of their lists. Complaints of this "favoritism" filled the nursing literature. Nursing superintendents exercised considerable control over hiring special-duty nurses for hospital patients, requesting their own graduates and taking special care to send work to their "pets" among the alumnae. Registries operated by individuals outside the hospital could be even more idiosyncratic. In one extreme example, where the registry was located in a boarding house filled with nurses, a seasoned resident warned a newcomer about the older nurses' stringent standards of dress and decorum; if they disapproved, they convinced the registrar not to call the nonconformist for cases. Informal hiring networks could help a nurse with ties to the community or the hospital, but they could also become the vehicles for a petty and arbitrary exclusivity.[7]

The economic arrangements of private duty constrained nurses' control at work and undermined their skills. Referred by doctors and paid by their patients, private-duty nurses were more directly vulnerable to their clientele than salaried hospital or public-health nurses. The organization of private duty locked nurses into relationships of personal service: physicians' authority and patients' caprices interfered with nurses' ability to define their own work. To keep herself at work, the freelancer had to satisfy doctors and patients according to standards that might be remote from her training school's definition of good nursing.

Although private-duty nurses had limited contact with doctors on the job, their medical colleagues could exert powerful leverage over their careers. A doctor who disliked a nurse's methods, her suggestions, or even her personality could dismiss her, might refuse to call her again, and could even get her informally blacklisted in the community. Such conditions severely constrained nurses' performance and initiative on the job. Nurses who found themselves working with unethical or incompetent doctors could intervene only at considerable risk to their own futures. Whether in the isolated situation of home duty or behind closed doors in a private hospital room, the nurse could not easily appeal to outside arbitrators in conflicts with doctors. Unlike the public-health nurse, who worked with a medical and lay board and often with other nurses, or the hospital nurse, who was surrounded by other workers and protected by bureaucratic channels, the private-duty nurse was the sole observer and judge of the doctor's practice. Under such circumstances, nurses' new claims to expertise could have little weight against established medical authority and doctors' unconstrained power.[8]

Hired by her patient and attending only one person at a time, the private nurse also had to shape her practice to lay standards. Wealthy and middle-class patients especially threatened the nurse's skills and craft pride. Such patients were unlikely to appreciate the fine points of a nurse's technique, or the skill involved in scrupulous observation. They often slighted the nurse's technical and scientific abilities to emphasize her personal characteristics and social demeanor. In letters to nursing journals, patients complained about their nurses' table manners, reading voices, appearances, or conversational facility. Prescriptive literature tacitly acknowledged the burden of such extraneous standards; one manual admitted, "The personality of the individual woman. . . . not infrequently goes for more than skill and devotion in the nursing itself."[9]

Some of the complaints that home patients made simply reflected understandable anxiety about an outsider invading the household and disrupting domestic routines. No doubt sick patients and their nervous relatives were especially sensitive to indiscretions. One household wrote *Trained Nurse and Hospital Review* to complain about a nurse who had treated the patient kindly but irritated other family members for a variety of offenses: she left wet towels on doorknobs, walked noisily, banged bedpans, smeared oil on the woodwork, and left fingermarks on doors and shades. An experienced patient rated several of her nurses in a letter to the same journal. One failed in the patient's regard by scattering powder around and not rinsing the tub after the patient's bath. She disliked another nurse for being *too* efficient. This nurse upset her patient by closing and stacking magazines that the woman preferred to scatter around the room.[10] While nursing manuals and journals stressed alertness to the patient's preference, even the most circumspect nurse could not avoid occasional lapses: an extra person in the household inevitably created some tension.

Patients' complaints often reflected a clear class bias as well, and nursing manuals and patients' letters instructed private-duty nurses in the innumerable details of correct appearance and behavior. One advised nurses to strive for "a well-bred, dignified demeanor," and specifically warned against "lounging, leaning on furniture, carrying the hands on the hips, staring, snuffing, and various other habits" no doubt too heinous to name. The author of another manual railed against habits and styles "typical of a certain class of Americans," including "untidy hair, body odor, vulgar cuts of the neck and skirt of the uniform, rolled hose, grotesque make-up, nail polish and chewing gum." One patient condemned his nurse for the "excruciating habit" of clearing her throat when preparing the patient's lunch in the kitchen; the sound carried upstairs and reportedly ruined the patient's appetite. As if this were not enough, the nurse was guilty of a further crime, this one clearly premeditated: with unacceptable insouciance, she picked her teeth "right in front of the patient, with a pin which she kept for the purpose in the front hem of her waist." In hospitals, nursing superintendents enforced similar standards for student and staff nurses, and nursing schools sought to instill "breeding" along with technical skills. But while hospital staff nurses might have to pass muster with their superintendents, their patients no longer had the economic leverage to demand conformity to particular social behavior.[11]

Private-duty patients exercised their prerogatives as employers to set and enforce exacting social standards. One patient complained of his nurse, "She could not carry on an intelligent conversation." In deference to the standards of genteel private-duty patients, manuals, nursing journals, and didactic fiction extolled the "cultured nurse." A survey published in the 1930s contained a cautionary tale about a sensitive convalescent doctor who claimed that his private-duty nurse had precipitated a relapse because she mispronounced so many words while reading aloud. Fiction carried the same message. Even the usually confident Cherry Ames quailed on private duty, wishing she had kept up on her reading. "For her patient was a brilliant man, and he demanded that his nurse, who was his constant companion, have a well-stocked mind." An anecdote in an ethics book underscored the rigorous social requirements of private duty. A doctor attending a private case in a hotel felt pleased with the nurse's service, so he asked her to dinner one evening. But in those telling close quarters, their relationship took an ominous turn. "His complacency gradually changed to acute discomfort and chagrin as he watched her lack of ease and her appalling ignorance of the rudiments of good table manners." The next day, he stormed into the school that had graduated her, "declaring that he considered it little short of criminal to send out a girl to earn a living, as a nurse must, so little prepared for close association with ordinary, well-behaved men and women."[12]

Other patients treated their nurses like domestic servants, asking them to mend, iron, cook, scrub, do laundry, and attend children in any free moment. As one private-duty nurse complained, "Many patients seem to think they are 'getting their money's worth' only if they keep the nurse running all the time, regardless of the fact that she is removed from her patient when doing these chores."[13] Every manual on private-duty nursing offered guidance on this difficult issue, and nurses on the job developed a variety of ingenious ways to resist household tasks and to draw clearer boundaries to define nurses' special skills. Still, they had only limited resources in a market where "untrained" nurses would happily replace them and in a situation where old-fashioned physicians sometimes sided with their patients, who had considerable control. As one manual advised bluntly, "To succeed in nursing one must give some satisfaction to the family regardless of their unreasonableness."[14]

Nurses ran into other conflicts with those below them in the class structure of the household, for servants often resented these intruders into the domestic hierarchy. Nurses' relationships with servants were notoriously difficult. As outsiders in a household already disorganized by illness, nurses did create extra work and introduce unfamiliar routines, and this alone might make them a focus for servants' resentments. Other nurses may have offended servants by their efforts to dissociate themselves from domestic work, or alienated household workers by officious airs. One nurse suggested that servants were indignant about waiting on nurses, who were themselves household employees; nurses earned higher wages and appeared to be doing less work.[15]

In defining the nurse's place in the private patient's home, the manuals balanced precariously between maintaining professional dignity and deferring to the social superiority of wealthy patients. Carefully defining the nurse's intermediate status in the household, they advocated a dignified distance from both family and servants. "The nurse who expects to be invited to take her meals with the family is as unsophisticated as one who consents to be classed with the servants," one pronounced. Another agreed, "A nurse is entirely justified in refusing to go to the kitchen for meals with the servants, but is she always justified in demanding that she be treated as a guest in the home?" The nurse who followed these prescriptions led a lonely life on duty, excluded from both the sociability of the kitchen and the intimacy of family life.[16]

On the job and off duty, the isolation of private duty haunted many nurses, as their memoirs reveal. The young woman left the camaraderie and reassuring order of the hospital to live and work alone. One nurse remembered scrambling for her first case to pay for a place to live. "Now I was 'on my own,' and I was completely at sea." Another memoir summed up private duty in a stark chapter titled "Isolation." She too recalled the sad transition from school life to freelance work. "I felt like a lost sheep, not to return to the hospital after each case." A nurse resuming private duty after military service in World War I exclaimed, "How one misses the comradeship of life over there," and manuals acknowledged the deprivation of the nurse working without the support and company of colleagues. The unpredictable hours of private duty disrupted sociability outside work as well. One nurse wrote plaintively, "People are too busy to bother to keep up friendship with a person who is never able to say her time is her own."[17]

Finally, freelance work could be devastatingly insecure. Private duty was seasonal, with work abundant in the winter months and less available in the healthier seasons of summer and fall.[18] Nurses chafed at the imposed idleness between cases and the anxious hours spent waiting for the registrar's call. Like other women workers, nurses needed their incomes; even before the depression, 53 percent of private-duty nurses were responsible for partial or full support of one or more dependents.[19] In slack seasons, or if the nurse herself became ill, she was thrown on her own limited resources.

By the 1920s, the disadvantages of private duty loomed large for most freelance nurses. Signs of spreading unemployment quickly dispelled concern about a postwar nursing shortage, and the touted freedom of freelancing became for many nurses a grim mockery as they scrambled for work in an overcrowded market. Each month, more local nursing associations or registries posted notices in the *American Journal of Nursing* to warn nurses that there was no work in their towns and cities.[20] Deepening unemployment strained the individual accommodations that private-duty nurses could make in the timing and performance of their work.

The professional associations faced the "private-duty problem" with growing concern. The intensive study that culminated in 1928 with the Burgess report revealed the economic and social dimensions of the crisis. As hospital schools multiplied between 1890 and 1920, their graduates swelled the ranks of private duty. Despite strenuous efforts, nursing leaders had been unable to check this expansion. The continuing stream of graduates had saturated the private-duty market. Between 1920 and 1930, the total number of trained nurses doubled, while the United States' population increased only 16 percent.[21] Other developments narrowed private duty's potential clientele. New funding for public-health or visiting nurses' agencies replaced the old individual charitable funding that had formerly provided poorer patients with private-duty nurses. Private-duty nurses' rising wages put their services out of the reach of many middle-class patients, and those who still hired a nurse often economized by using her for just a few days rather than retaining her throughout convalescence. Problems of distribution compounded the squeeze of a shrinking clientele and expanding workforce: the concentration of private-duty nurses in urban areas increased local competition for a limited number of patients.[22] A changing market dictated a stop to apprenticeship training, hospitals' reliance on student staffs, and the resulting proliferation of graduates from hospital schools.

The impact of these changes could be read in the lives of thousands of private-duty nurses. The Burgess report documented in rich detail the harsh working conditions and economic marginality of private-duty nurses. By every measure, freelance nurses suffered in comparison to their colleagues in hospital or public-health work. They worked longer hours. While most hospital staff nurses had twelve-hour duty by the end of the 1920s, and public-health nurses enjoyed a forty-two-hour week, 56 percent of private duty home cases kept nurses on duty for twenty-four hours. Even in the hospital, some 12 percent of private-duty nurses reported that they worked around the clock. Under these pressures, they also lost more days to fatigue and illness. They earned about seven dollars per shift, which compared favorably with other nurses' and other women's wages at first glance. But because of the irregular scheduling of their work, they earned considerably less over a year than public-health nurses, and slightly less than even their underpaid sisters in hospital jobs. Accumulated experience or extra education did not pay off in increased income.[23]

Moreover, their limited earnings had to buy more. Unlike hospital nurses, who lived in the nursing residence and got free food, laundry, and housing, private-duty nurses shouldered the expenses of maintaining a home. Their overhead was higher: they had to launder their own uniforms and pay their transportation to cases. A telephone might be optional for others, but for the private-duty nurse it was almost a necessity, because without it she might miss calls for work. Many private-duty nurses lived uncomfortably close to the margin of economic insecurity. Compared to other nurses in the Burgess report, they generally had less money in savings, and were more likely to have to borrow to meet their expenses. Private-duty nurses in the 1920s were, as one editorial suggested, "the Cinderellas of the nursing family."[24]

An anonymous account, "The Life Story of One Private Duty Nurse," helps to flesh out the statistics with a rare and carefully detailed description of one freelancer's earnings and expenses. She had three years of college education, more than most of her peers in private duty, and sixteen years of experience. In 1926, her best year since her graduation in 1910, she had made $1,203, slightly under the average reported in the Burgess survey. She had worked only 190 days, with 51 days of vacation and 118 passed waiting for new cases. In twelve months she had cared for 41 different patients, reflecting the general movement to shorter cases. Her longest assignment had lasted just twelve days. After paying for her small room and meeting other expenses, she ended with a deficit of over $100. Sympathetic to the plight of freelancers, the *American Journal of Nursing* presented the case as an illustration of the tightening economy of private duty.[25]

Yet a closer look at private-duty nurses' incomes suggests certain qualifications to the stark picture drawn in the Burgess report and in "The Life Story." Clearly freelancers occupied an ignominious position within nursing; they were deprived by comparison to other nurses. But compared to the labor force as a whole, private-duty nurses still commanded a respectable income. Even under the precarious conditions of a slipping market, their average annual income was $1,300, which, in 1929, placed them within the category of subsistence income for a family of five ($1,100–$1,400). In the same year,

42.4 percent of all families made less than $1,500. These figures must be interpreted cautiously. First, 43 percent of private-duty nurses had no records of their income—an intriguing fact in itself—so Burgess's average may be misleadingly high or low. Second, it is impossible to assess how much discretion private-duty nurses could exercise in their spending, since 53 percent did have at least partial responsibility for one or more dependents. Still, the comparison suggests that, as single wage-earners, private-duty nurses may have occupied a relatively privileged position.[26]

Other factors may have contributed to the sense of deprivation and economic insecurity expressed by so many private-duty nurses. Not knowing how much work they could get, freelancers must have had difficulty budgeting their incomes, and felt constrained about discretionary spending. In the flourishing consumer economy of the 1920s, nurses might well have felt a nagging sense of deprivation as they weighed the inducements of radios, cars, movies, or cosmetics against the need to save money as a hedge against slack times. "The Life Story" supports this interpretation; although the author's income seemed to compare favorably with that of other workers, it was not enough to meet expenses. This nurse also might well have felt deprived by comparison with others of her educational level: no doubt she hoped for and expected more than subsistence living. Still, like Burgess's average private-duty nurse, she was probably not poor by the general standards of the 1920s.

Evidence exists that some private-duty nurses lived in the grip of real poverty. A New York private-duty nurse wrote Burgess, "What are we going to do? For nearly three months I lived on one meal a day."[27] One unusual memoir documents a grim story of economic scarcity. In her last year of training school, Iva Marie Lowry contracted tuberculosis, one of the special hazards of hospital life. After graduation, she struggled to keep working to support her "very poor family." Her memoir documents a day-to-day struggle for survival. Lowry was driven from case to case, and sometimes from town to town, as indignant patients and doctors discovered her illness and fired her. Her limited income barely sufficed when she could work, but she collapsed periodically from exhaustion, undernourishment, and exacerbations of her disease. She faced her fulminating tuberculosis alone. In one bleak scene, she was overtaken by a tell-tale fit of coughing when attending a case. The relief nurse stood by coldly as the patient's daughter ordered Lowry out of the house. Gasping for breath, she got to a train station, where she sat alone until she revived somewhat from what she realized was a collapsed lung. She fled to another city for a short stint of work in a proprietary hospital run by a thoroughly unprincipled doctor. Finally she reached a sanatorium, where she received desperately needed medical care and then got a job. Although her story was surely not typical, it did underscore the frightening insecurity that could befall less fortunate private-duty nurses.[28]

As the unstable prosperity of the 1920s collapsed, more nurses crossed the line between relative and absolute deprivation. The depression years erased any ambiguity about nurses' economic position, as freelancers plunged into a situation of desperate scarcity. Private duty was increasingly defined as a discretionary expense, even a luxury, and as middle-class families cut back, the bottom dropped out of the private-duty market. By 1934, a Women's Bureau survey found that nurses' incomes had been slashed to about $500, placing nurses in the lowest fifth of family and single persons' incomes. In 1934, only one in four freelance nurses worked twenty days a month or more. By 1936, the journals noted improvement, but two out of three nurses still worked less than twenty days a month.[29]

Private duty would never regain its preeminence. The serious oversupply of nurses was only one of the many forces undermining this organization of work. As the "private-duty crisis" of the 1920s dragged on into the 1930s and 1940s, it became clear that the freelance market was not depressed, it was collapsing beyond reconstruction. Changes in consumer patterns reduced patient demand for nurses, even as the rise in

hospital use, changing hospital management and organization, and new medical technology made the skills and structure of private duty obsolete. Private-duty nurses' autonomy,
already limited, was steadily eroded by conditions beyond the
control of individual nurses or informal hospital and community networks.

Larger changes in medical care modified the content and
workplace of private-duty nursing. Associated with the new
skills and knowledge of scientific medicine, nursing had become more clearly defined as skilled work by 1920. New
patterns in private-duty practice reflected both the increasing
use of hospital care and the growing division of labor and
specialization in nursing. Private-duty nurses followed their
acutely ill patients to the hospital, leaving less specialized
home care to "practical" nurses. By 1921, the transition from
home to hospital workplace was already well underway: registries reported that about half of their cases were nursed in the
hospital. By the end of the decade, 80 percent of private-duty
nurses attended their cases in hospitals. Home care persisted,
but more and more it became the province of nurses who had
not taken the full hospital course. A 1943 survey indicated that
90 percent of the home cases were attended by such workers,
known as practical nurses, subsidiaries, auxiliaries, or "short-
course" nurses. As long chronic cases, convalescences, and
many obstetrical cases passed to practicals, trained nurses
worked harder on short cases with sicker patients.[30]

On the surface, one might expect this new division of
labor to boost the technical content of private-duty nursing
and to enhance its reputation as skilled work. Trained nurses
had gained a gratifying acceptance from most of the medical
profession by the mid-1920s, and the advantages of that legitimacy showed in hiring practices that favored the trained nurse
over her self-taught sister. Burgess's survey revealed that 84
percent of doctors recommended trained nurses over practicals for their private-duty cases, giving the graduate a stronger
position in the freelance market.[31] The shift to the hospital
workplace would seemingly secure the place of the trained

nurse. Hospital cases were more consistently demanding: acute care required technical skills that were clearly beyond the abilities of most laywomen. As important, the hospital workplace enforced the distinction between the nurse's special skills and the work done by domestic servants or laywomen in the family. In the hospital, private-duty nurses escaped the demands of the patient's household, and could restrict their duties more closely to actual bedside nursing.

But overall, the growing specialization of medicine and nursing eroded the skills and status of private-duty practice relative to hospital or public-health work. The working conditions and the organization of private duty limited nurses' opportunities to keep up with medical and nursing innovations. Isolated in their patients' homes or set apart in private hospital rooms, private-duty nurses had little chance to use new equipment or to observe the latest techniques. The unregulated freelance market offered no incentive for nurses to take postgraduate courses: they were understandably reluctant to spend time and money on further training that would not result in raises or promotions. As hospitals and public-health agencies began to hire more selectively, the least-educated nurses fled to the private-duty market. In turn, private duty became identified as a haven for nurses with fewer credentials, reinforcing the image of private duty as less skilled work.[32]

Changes in hospital use and management also made private-duty nurses increasingly marginal. In hospitals staffed by attendants or student nurses, private doctors had routinely recommended private-duty or "special" nurses for their sickest patients. But by the mid-1930s, hospitals had begun to hire graduates to supplement the student staffs. As the level of general care improved, the need for special-duty nurses lessened. Before World War I, lingering prejudices made patients reluctant to go to the hospital: the care and attention of a trained nurse had been invaluable in saving home patients with dreaded contagious diseases like typhoid, scarlet fever, or diphtheria. Through the 1920s, as hospital use increased and more women began to give birth in hospitals, the special nurse often simply duplicated services already provided by the hospital staff. With increasing efforts to rationalize hospital work and a general preoccupation with efficiency in other industries, observers of nursing services grew critical of private duty. Having one nurse care for just one patient seemed a waste of skilled labor. Increasingly, the private-duty nurse came to be seen as a luxury rather than a necessary adjunct to hospital care.

II. THE SEARCH FOR STABILITY

Nursing leaders responded to the private-duty crisis with sweeping proposals for a reorganization that would assert the structural control of work that characterizes a profession. The professional associations addressed private-duty nurses' problems mostly through the removed and long-term strategy of restricting access to the profession. They redoubled their efforts to raise standards and to limit the numbers of graduates through control of nursing education. Contemporary accounts in journals and surveys repeatedly emphasized the link between apprenticeship training and private-duty unemployment. With less enthusiasm, they worked to organize and regulate private-duty practice. But it quickly became evident that leaders had few plans and little motivation for resuscitating private duty as the major form of nursing practice. Embracing the imperatives of rationalization, and socially distant from their less-educated freelance colleagues, leaders did little to support the unfortunate women caught in private duty's demise. Rather, they looked beyond individuals to plan for nursing's future as a restructured and rationalized occupation centered in the hospital.

Leaders tried half-heartedly to organize private nurses to exercise a de facto professional self-regulation. On a local level, they advised freelancers to form "official" or "central" registries, run by graduate nurses according to standards set by the professional associations. Through these agencies, leaders hoped to bring the community's nursing services under nurses' control, gradually replacing hospital or commercial registries as they demonstrated the superiority of registries run by "professional" standards. Self-consciously echoing the service orientation characteristic of the professions, proponents argued that such registries would enable nurses to provide more efficient and thorough service to the community. The same centralized nursing network, of course, would also join competing registries, institutions, and public-health agencies into a unified body that could act in nurses' concerted interests. One supporter wrote, "This registry might act as the hub around which all nursing interests might develop, and we do not yet know its possibilities."[33]

Through the plan for central registries, professional leaders tried to fit private duty into the mold of professional aspirations. As Eliot Freidson has argued, the professional's independence in practice is attained through close regulation of the market and defended by the group's control over conditions of practice. The free access to the private-duty market and the absence of uniform standards indicated the gap between nursing leaders' aspirations and their very limited power. With central registries, nurses could exert more control over nursing practice in the community and define the kind of nursing that patients received. "Practicals" could be restricted to certain cases, or excluded altogether. Nursing cases could be assigned on the basis of each nurse's technical abilities and experience, replacing the local control of hospital and commercial registries with rational, uniform standards set by a professional group. Proposals for central registries also sought to establish nurses' exclusive authority over nursing care, as they stipulated that all requests for nurses should be channelled through the official registries.[34]

Few central registries were actually started. While the journals offer only scattered information about the fate of the plan, its failure is hardly mysterious. Organizers of registries faced overwhelming odds with few concrete resources. In a highly competitive market, they did not have the legal leverage of mandatory licensing or the advantage of consistent and reliable support from doctors. Moreover, the success of central registries depended on a degree of consensus and a level of national self-organization that nurses simply had not achieved. In this context, attempts to assert broad control over nursing services were largely futile. Where nurses did start official registries, many probably suffered the predictable fate of newcomers to an already overcrowded market. One nurse offered intriguing evidence of the marginal position of the official registry in her community. She wrote to *Trained Nurse* to complain that she had had trouble even finding a central registry, because many of the local hospitals did not use the nurse-managed service. In a competitive market, the central registry could not keep up with better-established employment bureaus. The nurse reported that she had received only one five-day case in twelve weeks on call with the official registry. When she finally switched to a commercial registry, she got eight weeks of work during the next twelve weeks.[35]

Perhaps, too, the registries met active resistance from doctors, nurses, and patients, who all felt they had more control in the informal networks of "nonofficial" registries. Predictably, doctors opposed any erosion of their own prerogative to choose and direct nurses, and patients may also have preferred a system that could bend to their individual choices. Private-duty nurses themselves had reasons to doubt the benefits of rationalization. Undoubtedly, many felt threatened by leaders' eagerness to introduce a system of ranking in private duty. Given the American Nurses' Association's history and commitments, such a hierarchy was likely to emphasize educational credentials and to discount experience. As the nursing group with the least formal education, private-duty nurses were not likely to embrace such a plan. When the ANA attempted a national placement service in 1931, it required participating nurses to have four years of high school education, and charged a placement fee. Five years later, only 581 nurses were registered. The required standards for placement, *Trained Nurse* speculated, "may have caused some antagonism on the part of graduates who were barred from registering and on the part of hospitals which maintained the same standards." For whatever reasons, official registries and placement services never gained the dominant market position they needed to control nursing practice effectively.[36]

The American Nurses' Association also supported two other interim solutions for freelance nurses, "group nursing" and "hourly nursing." Both were efforts to revive a broader middle-class market for private duty. In group nursing, one special nurse attended two or three patients in adjoining hospital rooms, an arrangement midway between the old one-to-one relationship of private duty and the general care available from hospital staff nurses. Supporters of the plan hoped that dividing the cost of private duty among several patients would make it a desirable alternative for patients of moderate means. Hourly nursing followed a similar logic. Under this plan, the private nurse would make rounds to a number of home patients, each of whom needed only a few hours of skilled care.[37] In theory, this sort of coordination and rationalization of care probably did have some potential for expanding the clientele of private duty. But to most private-duty nurses, it looked suspiciously like a scheme to use fewer workers to cover the same number of cases. In their immediate and desperate need for employment, few private-duty nurses could afford to trade existing work for the uncertain long-term hope of expanding their market. One nurse wrote to describe the acute shortage of work in her city, and exclaimed, "Why under these conditions try to figure out a way to fix it so we have still less work?" On the job, the disadvantages to individual nurses were obvious. Both plans accelerated the pace of work, and hourly nursing involved extra transportation costs and uncompensated time in between appointments. Under such circumstances, private-duty nurses could hardly be expected to share leaders' enthusiasm for the greater efficiencies of group and hourly nursing.[38]

Both leaders and their critics tried to use the professional association as a vehicle for private-duty nurses' self-organization, exhorting freelancers to join special sections within the state and national nursing associations. As the official organ of the American Nurses' Association, *AJN* urged freelancers to use these groups to define uniform standards—in practice, to ratify leaders' suggested standards. Acutely aware of the ANA's low membership, leaders worked to recruit more nurses to establish a stronger national organization and a more unified occupation. *Trained Nurse* was consistently wary of nursing's official leadership, and it maintained a strong focus on private-duty nurses long after the ANA had tacitly abandoned them. Strongly identified with private-duty nurses and sensitive to their growing marginality, the editors of *Trained Nurse* encouraged private nurses to fight for their rightful place in the ANA and to compel leaders to represent their interests.[39]

Despite such recruitment efforts, private-duty nurses kept their distance from the professional organizations. Although private-duty nurses constituted a clear plurality of working nurses until 1940, they never exerted proportionate influence in the professional associations. Even in state nursing associations where private-duty nurses dominated the membership rolls, many did not attend meetings or otherwise participate in the groups' activities. Nursing leaders and their critics both despaired of mobilizing this seemingly passive constituency.[40]

The conditions and structure of private duty posed real barriers to organization. Most simply, the unpredictable timing and long hours of private-duty cases restricted nurses' ability to participate in any voluntary associations. The work setting and freelance practice of private-duty work also limited group activity and collective sentiments. In their isolation, private-duty nurses often had no regular contact with their colleagues, and as the market became increasingly competitive, encounters at registries or in hospital corridors became less likely to engender a spirit of friendly cooperation. The intense localism of private-duty nurses posed another formidable obstacle. The tight circles of nurses from the same schools or communities did not yield easily to the more impersonal organization of state or national associations: personal loyalties outweighed the abstract notion of professional loyalties. As one author acknowledged, "nurses until very recently . . . have been terribly snobbish. They held up their noses at women from other schools or states. Much good comradeship has been lost for this [reason]."[41] By circumstance and by tradition, the private-duty nurse was an individualist and often a loner.

The organization of private duty also set freelancers apart from other nurses. Private-duty nurses and public-health nurses were not likely to meet on the job or even in professional associations; public health nurses had their own active organization. Special duty in hospitals permitted some contact between private-duty nurses and students or graduates on hospital staffs, but conflict often ran high between the two groups. The *American Journal of Nursing* acknowledged that "there is sometimes an attitude on the part of the student body that special nurses are a necessary evil," and Burgess noted with restraint: "Apparently the relationship between special duty nurses and the other workers in the hospital is not always a happy one." Both staff nurses and supervisors were likely to see freelancers as interlopers. Specials used the common supplies of the floor, and sometimes depended on staff nurses for relief or assistance during their shifts. Yet because they were paid to attend the patient full-time, they could not easily reciprocate. Their work routines and relatively unsupervised practice threatened the discipline and hierarchy of the hospital. Harassed hospital nurses resented the private-duty nurse's independence and more leisured pace, and often treated the special as an intruder, excluding her from the camaraderie and mutual aid of the floor. One private-duty nurse complained that a staff nurse had refused to help her move her moribund 200-pound patient; the struggling special was forced to enlist the patient's doctor to assist her with general bedside care. "These petty tyrannies are found in many hospitals," she concluded. Superintendents and staff nurses accused private-duty nurses of hoarding hospital supplies for their patients, appropriating linen for their own use, and carrying off hospital food to stock their own kitchens. Apparently fearful that the untrammeled freelancer might breed insubordination, superintendents enforced social distance: often they segregated students and specials in separate sitting rooms and dining facilities. On the whole, there was little to support the growth of a sense of common interests and identity.[42]

Although the arrangements of private duty kept some nurses away from professional associations by default, others apparently were voting with their feet. In rejecting the journals' pleas for participation, a few nurses revealed their disillusionment with the nursing organizations. Powerful local nurses sometimes silenced others by exercising autocratic control over the organizations. One private-duty nurse observed, "There is a definite connection between speaking up about things and getting work. If you have too many opinions you can't get work to do. So I keep still as well as I ever did." Another nurse resigned from her professional association in disgust after thirteen years of membership. She wrote *Trained Nurse* to explain: "Several times I tried to follow your advice and speak my piece at the district meetings. Let me tell you I learned then to shut up for I didn't get called to the hospital for work for weeks after each try. . . . I had to choose between bread and freedom of speech, and I chose bread." A letter with a happier conclusion showed the same conservative control in a California district association. A group of nurses repeatedly introduced a resolution in support of the eight-hour day for private duty, which was still not universal in 1940. "Always the Board of Directors or the committee killed it before we could take any definite action." At last the motion succeeded when determined supporters managed to pack the meeting.[43]

Such letters suggest the conflicts of interest that divided nurses. The ANA could not easily serve both supervisory nurses and their subordinates, and this problem would worsen as nurses moved from private duty into hospital staff jobs. Also, the professional aspirations that fueled the ANA generally led to an emphasis on long-term goals, with a concomitant lack of interest in short-term remedies. Freelancers may well have agreed with one critic who challenged *Trained Nurse*: "You ask what nurses want. Well, for one thing they want you to stop sticking up for the ANA. You think it can be made into an association that will fight for nurses as well as nursing. We think it is too late for that."[44]

Professional leaders apparently had little commitment to maintaining the freelance organization of private-duty nursing. By the mid-1920s, they considered private duty a lost cause, and they did little to improve existing conditions. When private-duty nurses took leaders at their word and tried to assume a more active role in the national ANA, they were edged aside. At the 1930 Biennial conference, the private duty section, a caucus in the national group, passed a resolution to have private-duty nurses represented on all standing committees. In 1931, a reader wrote to ask where these nurses were. The president of the ANA answered evasively, "It isn't always possible or desirable to change committee memberships." The maverick editor of *Trained Nurse* repeatedly flailed at the professional associations, criticizing leaders for ignoring private-duty nurses. In January 1937 she worried, "Is the Private Duty Nurse Standing Still?" and by March, the journal printed a letter with the headline, "Are We Embalmed?" Apparently unmoved, leaders seemed ready to bury the corpse as they turned their full energies to hospital-based nursing.[45]

III. RESOLUTE FREELANCERS: RESISTANCE ON THE JOB

Although private-duty nurses never found an effective voice in the nursing associations and never formed a national organization of their own, they were not passive in the face of a declining market. Even as larger changes in medical care were undercutting private duty, nurses themselves were struggling to redefine the content and social relationships of their work. Through the 1920s and 1930s, journals and surveys reveal two broad perspectives on private duty that challenged leaders' vision of hospital-based nursing. The first viewpoint, which was clearly a minority position by the 1920s, drew on the older identification of nursing with women's domestic roles. These nurses looked back to an image of a golden age of private duty, and bid others to do the same. Sometimes they identified themselves as old-timers, nurses who had graduated before World War I; other times they called themselves "old-fashioned." These were nursing's traditionalists, women who represented an older version of nursing rooted in the context of family and neighborhood. Just as they had recoiled from leaders' professional ideology, so they resisted efforts to rationalize private-duty nursing.

The second perspective, which many nurses shared, gathered impetus from the changing options and prescriptions for young women in the teens and 1920s. Comparing their work to other jobs available to women, they grew restive under the difficult conditions and constraining relationships of private duty. On the job, these nurses arranged their work to reduce the elements of personal service associated with private duty, and they used individual strategies to improve their working conditions. In many ways, their view of nursing's problems coincided with leaders' analyses. But they resisted the move to hospital-based nursing, staunchly defending their prerogatives as freelance workers. They were individualists, resistant to traditional claims and leery of the control of institutional employers.

At first glance, the traditional perspective seems no more than the jeremiads of a few moralistic souls. These nurses saw the problems of private duty as a moral crisis and called for "a reawakening, a real religion, a reconsecration." "What Does She Want?" one article inquired rhetorically, and answered emphatically, "She wants to *gain* more *spiritual comfort*, from her service to the sick. It is *wrong* to feel that commercial gain seems all that is worth while. In this way lies chaos!" Grandly above venal considerations, this rhetoric demonstrated little grasp of the economic realities of private duty. For most nurses, unemployment decisively undercut the glories of self-sacrifice, and a secure income undoubtedly loomed large in their view of spiritual comfort.[46]

A clearly discernable social and cultural context supported the traditional nurses' praise of private duty. At a time when most nurses were striving to define nursing with reference to scientific knowledge and technical skills, traditional nurses described their work in personal and emotional terms. As one wrote, "When I enter a home to care for the sick I like to meet and know all the family. I want to go deep down in their hearts and stay with them." For these nurses, the lines between work and social life blurred, and nursing defined not their employment so much as their place in the community. Many reported "cases" that extended into a continuing involvement with the patient and family. One nurse told of meeting an old patient in the dime store and immediately getting an invitation to dinner. "Now that's what happens to a private nurse. We have so many invitations that if we hope to continue practicing we are obliged to refuse them." A grateful patient wrote warmly of a nurse who had tended her five-year-old daughter through a bout of typhoid fever. "During those weeks . . . a friendship was made which will last through life, and if I were not living, our daughter would turn to her for the help, advice, and comfort that only a woman can give."[47]

On the longer cases that were once the staple of private duty, the nurse sometimes became more like a close friend or relative than an employee. One nurse and her female patient shared a common passion for travel; to fill the long hours of illness they pored over guidebooks and schedules to conjure up itineraries for perfect trips. After six months the patient died, leaving the nurse money and instructions to travel the itineraries they had mapped. Another nurse moved in to care for an 85-year-old woman and stayed until the woman's death ten years later. Describing this case, she remembered, "We had grown very fond of each other, and her going has left a great emptiness in my life." The obituary for an 1893 graduate commemorated an even longer association: "Miss Treglown

had been a private duty nurse and for forty years cared sym-
pathetically and tenderly for the same patient." These experiences reveal the real rewards that some nurses derived from
the code of selfless service, the personal intimacy and the
close-knit communities that sustained their work.[48]

Perhaps only a few private-duty nurses ever lived in the
world these anecdotes evoke, and by the 1920s it was clearly
lost to most nurses. Certainly it was beyond the reach of
moral fervor alone, the only "solution" that traditional nurses
ever proposed. Their protests sounded an anachronistic note
in the 1920s, as they themselves wryly acknowledged in their
pessimistic views of the modern spirit. Younger nurses impa-
tiently rejected the traditionalists' earnest sense of mission,
discarding the moral imperatives of women's culture for the
individual rewards and "self-fulfillment" of a new age.
"Women are not willing to be subjugated any longer. The
nurse is crying out for justice, for a bit of the sun and fun as
well as the other women." In this context, the pious exhortations of traditional nurses seemed senseless, even neurotic.
"Where is the normal person who likes always to give and
never receive?" one modern demanded.[49]

Traditionalists had no answers to the questions of this
new age, and they could not understand these women's impatience to claim their places as skilled workers. The isolation
of their stance marks the distance that nursing had come from
domestic duty to skilled paid work. At the same time, in a
curious way, theirs was the most radical challenge to the
rationalization of nursing. They clung to a view of work that
rejected a narrow contractual model. For them, womanly
service transcended the market relationships of nursing-for-
hire: paid work was informed by and interpreted within older
economies of obligation and reciprocity.

Caught in the economic relationships that traditionalists
deplored, most nurses experienced deep dissatisfaction with
private duty. The complaints underscored the growing constraints of the work, and, at the same time, signaled private-
duty nurses' changing consciousness of themselves as workers

and as women. Their training and work generated a pride in their craft. They had experienced hospitals' urgency to recruit student nurses; they had worked in the aura of medicine's rising prestige; they had heard teachers, supervisors, and nursing leaders wax eloquent about the dignity of the professional nurse. Such experiences bolstered nurses' sense of themselves as skilled workers, entitled to a more secure social and economic position. Meanwhile, the larger social environment of young nurses fostered other new expectations that lent added bitterness to the difficulties of private duty. The growing possibilities for women's white-collar work and the insistent appeal of advertising and mass media gave a false sense of expansiveness to the teens and 1920s, a glittering prosperity that posed a galling contrast to the private-duty nurse's straitened position. Both work and social settings supported new claims on the job, and, within the increasing limits of private duty, nurses still acted to defend their prerogatives as skilled workers.

Aggrieved nurses repeatedly compared their wages and working conditions to other women's occupations. "Let us not be so meek and uncomplaining . . . but stand for the recognition of the merits of the professional woman. . . . We cannot afford to underbid the domestic if we are not prepared to fulfill our contract." Citing the long hours, fatigue, and isolation of the work, a California nurse concluded, "A private duty nurse lives a slave's life. . . . Any washerwoman earns 50 cents an hour." A nurse from Washington noted, "All other women's work is eight hours, while ours is twenty-four." These women decisively rejected the rhetoric of self-sacrifice and demanded a social life separated from their work. "There is no more reason why a nurse should kill herself working at her profession and not be able to have any time for social life than a schoolteacher or stenographer should," one nurse insisted. Even one relatively satisfied nurse was acutely aware of the contrast between nursing and other women's jobs. "I have never been sorry that nursing has been my life's work," she wrote after twenty-seven years in private duty. "It has given me much, but financially I am far behind other women of my age who started life in other fields of endeavor, teachers, stenographers, bookkeepers, saleswomen, etc."[50]

Burgess's survey revealed the extent of private-duty nurses' dissatisfaction: 45 percent of freelancers wanted to leave their field, compared to 14 percent of public-health nurses and 18 percent of hospital nurses. Among younger and better-educated private-duty nurses, discontent ran even higher: 57 percent of nurses who had graduated in the last five years, and 62 percent of the nurses with college degrees, planned to quit. One nurse wrote, "I will land in the poorhouse at my present mode of living. I hope to go back to secretarial work, the work I did before becoming a nurse." In a written memoir, another nurse explained her decision to give up private duty and enroll in a clerical course.[51] There is no way of knowing how many nurses did leave for other jobs, but the large number who planned to quit may help to explain the relative lack of organization among unhappy private-duty nurses. A worker with one foot out the door is not likely to undertake the arduous task of organizing for broad, but also elusive, remedies.

Social relationships on the job added insult to the injuries of low wages and difficult working conditions. The changing composition of the private-duty market widened the class differences between nurses and their patients. After 1920, the average private-duty patient was more likely to be from the upper-middle or upper classes, that species of patient most threatening to the private nurse's self-respect and autonomy at work. Qualitative sources and surveys suggest the narrowing clientele of private nursing by the 1920s. Autobiographies from the late nineteenth and early twentieth centuries describe a variety of private-duty workplaces. One nurse slept on the floor where she cared for two diphtheria patients in a shack with no running water; nursed three prostitutes through the measles in a quarantined brothel; attended a typhoid case on an isolated ranch; and then stayed with a rich woman convalescing in an elegant home.[52] By the 1920s, similar accounts in

journals and manuals depict wealthy patients almost exclusively: the diverse clientele of private duty apparently had
disappeared. Available surveys confirm this impression.
Burgess found that growing numbers of patients felt they
could not afford private nursing services. At the end of the
1930s, an American Medical Association survey found that
families with annual incomes under $1,500, or 60 percent of
the population, rarely used private nursing services. Most
patients came from only 10 percent of the population, those
families that earned over $3,000 a year.[53] In the homes of their
class superiors, nurses were most vulnerable to demands for
personal service and hard put to defend their own sense of
skill.

In her well-known short story "Horsie" (1925), humorist
Dorothy Parker satirizes bourgeois manners by drawing a
dramatic contrast between a drab spinster nurse and the Cru-
gers, her wealthy employers. The story captures the difficult
class relationships of private duty and signals the declining
status of the work in the social context of the 1920s. The nurse,
dubbed "Horsie" by the couple, spends five weeks in the
household caring for the spoiled wife after childbirth. "Miss
Wilmarth was an admirable trained nurse, sure and calm and
tireless, with a real taste for the arranging of flowers in bowls
and vases." These qualities make her the butt of the couple's
merciless humor; they mock her because nursing defines and
absorbs her. The demands of the job are presented as incom-
patible with private life and female sexuality. "She was tall,
pronounced of bone, erect of carriage; it was somehow impossible to speculate upon her appearance undressed. Her long
face was innocent, indeed ignorant, of cosmetics." Every
detail of her appearance is subordinated to her work, from her
severe knot of hair, "practical to support her little high cap,"
to her hands, "scrubbed and dry, with nails cut short."[54]

The worlds of marriage and upper middle-class life exclude her; she is an awkward third with the light-hearted
young couple. The veneer of "culture" that Parker satirizes in
Horsie's flower-arranging skills proves woefully deficient in

the revealing situations of home duty. Her profession earns her a place at the family table. "Everyone had always heard of trained nurses' bristling insistence that they not be treated as servants; Miss Wilmarth could not be asked to dine with the maids."[55] But she cannot match the careless sophistication of those born to the manner. At dinner, night after night, she betrays herself in vain attempts to imitate upper middle-class style. Her social isolation is complete. Her employer dreads the dinners and the servants resent her for her familiarity with the family. She leaves the case to return to her small apartment and the mother she supports, pathetically grateful for the flower that Mr. Cruger gives her as she says goodbye.

This portrayal of a bare life of undeserved loneliness shows private duty in the unflattering light of the new expectations of the 1920s. Private duty's traditional rewards are gone. In the asymmetrical class relationship of nurse and patient, real intimacy is impossible. Miss Wilmarth's work detaches her from any potential community of equals while also foreclosing the possibility of upward mobility. Frozen on the margins of social life, Miss Wilmarth lives an ascetic existence relieved only by her vicarious enjoyment of her patients' luxurious lives. Her devotion to duty and her efforts to perform in the appropriate social style make her foolish and pathetic. Absorbed in a role with such limited rewards, she loses even the defense of irony.

Unlike the innocent Horsie, many private duty nurses were intensely conscious of the power of class on the job, and eager to claim their own prerogatives as skilled workers. They worked vigorously to limit the social control of their class superiors and employers. Even in the harsh unemployment of the 1920s, many nurses defended their skills and their private lives by refusing to nurse home cases. Although only 2 percent of the nurses that Burgess surveyed admitted to registering against home cases, 40 percent of the registrars declared that they could not find nurses for home patients. As one complained, "Our nurses are most independent and want to choose their cases. They all want to nurse in the hospital." In another city, the registrar reported that favored alumnae or local nurses almost invariably refused home calls and waited for hospital special duty; only the more marginal "outside" nurses would work in patients' homes. Registrars commiserated over "this very trying and embarrassing condition" to no avail.[56]

The hospital environment tacitly enforced nurses' legitimacy as skilled workers. The visible apparatus of nursing and medicine underscored the nurse's skill to the layperson. In contrast to their uneasy patients, nurses were insiders, initiates into the esoteric technical and institutional workings of the hospital. The nurse's location in a specialized workplace revised the patient's class prerogatives: in hospitals, nurses gained social control over their patients. While the nurse at home had to claim a precarious niche for herself in the routines and social relationships of the household, the hospital special worked in an environment tailored to medical and nursing routines. At home, patients commanded their own range of resources to supplement or contravene the nurse's authority. Their cooks and laundresses knew their preferences; family members and friends were at hand to run errands, to entertain them, even to support them in rebellions against medical and nursing orders. Isolated in hospitals, patients relied on their nurses for access to institutional resources and to the outside world. The nurse alone brought meals and clean linen, took messages, screened visitors, and mediated medical directives. The private patient in the hospital still retained the final prerogative of an employer, and could dismiss an unsatisfactory nurse. But short of this last recourse, the hospital patient lost much of his or her former power to define the content and practice of the nurse's work.

By insisting on hospital special duty, young nurses struggled to preserve their old advantages as freelance workers and to assert a new independence on the job. In the specialized workplace of the hospital, they escaped many of the constraints of personal service and enjoyed better working conditions. At the same time, though, they rejected leaders' solution of institutional employment for nurses. Despite the stark data of private duty's declining economic position, nurses widely believed that freelancers earned more than hospital staff nurses.[57] As well, hospital staff nursing was regarded as only an apprenticeship, "students' work" that was beneath the dignity of a graduate nurse. Even in a narrowing market, many preferred to take their chances on uncertain freelancing rather than submit to the authority of a nursing superintendent and the rigid work and social discipline of their training school days. With hospital special duty, freelancers hoped to combine the advantages of private duty with many of the benefits of hospital employment.

But whether at home or in the hospital, freelance practice had no secure future. The depression accelerated the transformation of nursing, both in its devastating influence on the private-duty market and in the changes it wrought in the hospital industry. Hospitals' resistance to hiring graduates began to yield in the 1930s. Many smaller hospitals found that nursing schools were no longer economically advantageous, and turned to new sources of labor. Nursing school enrollments dropped, so that even hospitals with schools sometimes needed to supplement their staffs with graduates. Throughout the 1930s, hospitals' need for labor rose steadily as demand increased and new federal funding boosted hospital budgets.

Mobilization for World War II lent new impetus to the reorganization of nursing services. In August 1942, the *American Journal of Nursing* printed a letter that foreshadowed the fate of private duty, as patriotic fervor pressed forward the logic of rationalization. The author, a nurse, exhorted private-duty nurses to leave their work and join the war effort. "Private duty is a highly respected art—and a luxury, nearly always." Two months later, the American Nurses' Association officially adopted the same position, urging private nurses to relocate to hospital staffs or to volunteer for military service. By the end of 1943, the War Manpower Commission had classified private duty as non-essential service. Some pri-vate-duty nurses left freelance work for military service. For civilian nurses, the threat of a nurses' draft may have speeded the transition to hospital staff jobs, which were classified as essential. For the first time, more nurses worked on hospital staffs than in private duty.[58]

The trend continued into the postwar years. By 1948, three nurses worked on hospital staffs for every one in private duty. Few new graduates entered the field. The growing specialization of hospitals eroded private-duty nurses' skills. With the opening of intensive care units in the late 1950s, private duty lost its last solid claim to providing a technically specialized service. More and more, private duty came to be seen as nursing's backwater. Speaking in 1976, one graduate of the 1930s dismissed private duty altogether, briskly summing up her experience. "Park Avenue and Fifth Avenue patients. And you were like a servant . . . I just didn't feel like I was nursing."[59]

Although private duty was well outside the mainstream of nursing even by 1940, both traditionalists and individualists indirectly shaped nursing's future by resisting it. The histori-cal memory of private duty influenced the first generation of nurses working in the newly dominant hospital. General-duty nurses of the late 1930s and 1940s would invoke the ideal of the freelancer's autonomy to demand better working conditions, and would appeal to traditional conceptions of the nurse's relationship to her patient as they resisted scientific manage-ment in the hospital. Although private-duty nurses could not defend the freelance organization of nursing, the individ-ualists' new demands on the job and their clear conception of nursing as skilled work had largely replaced the traditional ideology of nursing as womanly service. Moved by these expectations, new generations of nurses would alter their relationships with doctors, patients, and hospital adminis-trators.

CHAPTER 4

Public-Health Nurses and the "Gospel of Health," 1920–1955

As private-duty nurses faced the steady decline of their market, public-health nurses were building a place for themselves in the setting of the expanding lay public-health reform movement. Trudging down city streets or jolting over country roads in their Fords, public-health nurses brought bedside nursing services to people who could not afford private duty, and solicited patients for the new services of preventive medicine. Like private-duty nurses, they often traveled to their patients, and most worked alone. But the organization of public-health services and their relative independence from mainstream medicine gave public-health nurses an unprecedented autonomy at work. Even as the skills and status of private duty eroded, public-health nurses claimed special expertise in the developing field of preventive medicine and established themselves as an elite corps within nursing.

Public-health reformers self-consciously marked the distance between their work and traditional curative medicine. Physicians' clientele was largely self-selected, and patients rarely solicited medical advice except when driven by unpleasant symptoms. For the most part, doctors limited themselves to curing disease or moderating its discomforts. Scornful of those humble aims, public-health reformers enthusiastically assumed the task of conquering disease altogether. Scientific medicine had revealed the "laws of health": an informed public had only to apply this wisdom to their daily lives. "Health flows from right living," one nurse explained. "It comes as a by-product of life that is wholesome, fine and full of opportunity for growth and function of natural body systems." With millennial optimism, participants in the public-health movement set new goals for medicine. "What are we working toward?" asked another nurse, and she answered buoyantly, "I see a new type of human being, strong, vigorous and virile, not merely free from disease but enjoying abundant health and vigor." United behind this new vision, public-health nurses tirelessly promoted the new services of preventive medicine to skeptical doctors and potential clients. In the process, they carved out a special place for themselves.[1]

The history of public-health nursing offers a glimpse of the possibilities available to nurses in a setting somewhat removed from the controlling influence of physicians. In public-health work, nurses developed a special identity and their own nursing method. Allied with reformers, they set themselves apart from their medical colleagues and from other nurses. The organization of public-health work provided an institutional form within which nurses' independence could flourish. Located on the fringes of mainstream medicine, public-health nurses worked in institutions that operated beyond the lengthening reach of the hospital and largely outside the control of the medical profession. On the job, they expanded the scope of nursing duties and responsibilities, acting with considerable independence even as they honored the formal line between nursing and medical prerogatives. More than either private-duty or hospital nurses, public-health nurses shook off their role as the physician's hand, to set out and act on their own sense of nursing's sphere and mission.

Public-health nurses would come closer than any other nurses to claiming the privileges of professionals. Their history would show the pleasures and opportunities of relatively unconfined work, which is the enduring attraction of the professions. It would also point to the limitations of professional ideology, its elitism and self-defeating exclusivity. Inspired with a mission of reform and the hubris of expert knowledge, public-health nurses sometimes grew insensitive to their clients. Proud of their separate place, public-health nurses could not make common cause with other nurses when they most needed that support. And in the end, as they found their autonomy undermined by their own successes in promoting preventive work, their history would confirm and clarify the limits imposed on nursing by medical professionalization.

I. "THE BOND OF A COMMON PURPOSE": ORIGINS AND IDEOLOGY

Coined in 1912, the term "public-health nursing" reflected an emerging sense of common identity among nurses working outside the usual contexts of private duty or hospital jobs. The mission of "positive health" linked nurses in visiting nurses' associations and settlement houses, child welfare and anti-venereal disease associations, factory dispensaries and department store clinics. The public-health movement of the early twentieth century drew its special character and ideology from a range of reform and medical activities, and nurses self-consciously claimed this diverse heritage as their own.

The professionalization of reform had created new opportunities for nurses well before public health became a recognized nursing specialty. The Women's Branch of the New York City Mission began to send out trained nurses for home visiting in 1877. In 1886, philanthropic women founded district nursing associations in Boston and Philadelphia, hiring nurses in place of the genteel laywomen who had traditionally visited the sick poor. In 1893, Lillian Wald and Mary Brewster linked nursing to Progressive reform, moving to New York's Lower East Side to live and work in what was soon known as the Nurses' Settlement. Other philanthropically supported nursing settlement houses opened in Los Angeles, San Francisco, and Orange, New Jersey, in 1897 and 1898. Identified with Progressive reform, nursing settlements were quick to expand their activities beyond care of the sick poor to other projects ranging from school nursing to labor organization. Both visiting nurses' associations and settlement houses gave nurses a niche in the developing apparatus of urban social services, and forged connections between nursing and reform movements in the cities.[2]

The sanitary movement was another important precedent for public-health nurses, moving reformers from moralism to pragmatic environmentalism. Consciousness of public health as an issue had developed throughout the nineteenth century, as growing cities faced problems of water supply, lighting, garbage removal, and housing. As epidemics swept through one city after another, concerned citizens worked to identify and control the sources of infection. Before the elaboration of the germ theory, many observers concluded that disease was spread by miasma, the unsalubrious airs exuded by garbage, open sewers, and overcrowded districts. Early public health initiatives thus focused on improving the urban environment, and the sanitary movement did help to limit the sources and spread of infection. Although public health turned in new directions as the germ theory gained acceptance, it never entirely lost the nineteenth-century movement's broad social definition of health.[3]

The institutions and agencies of public-health nursing took shape in the first two decades of the twentieth century. The germ theory, widely accepted by the late nineteenth century, spawned a number of lay organizations that took on the battle against single diseases. These associations offered new opportunities in preventive work. Anti-venereal disease campaigns stressed "health education" along with case-finding and treatment. Anti-tuberculosis associations underwrote other educational efforts: in 1904, a national organization opened chapters in Baltimore, Cleveland, and Chicago. At the same time, public-health reformers began to shift their attention from the larger urban environment to the more immediate setting of the home and family. Progressive reform steered public-health fervor toward an intense concern for child welfare. A 1909 White House conference produced disturbing data on infant and maternal mortality rates in the United States. In other efforts, Progressives investigated child labor and agitated for restraining legislation. The Children's

Bureau, founded in 1912 through Lillian Wald's influence, gave organizational form and tax funding to child welfare services.[4]

Nurses also organized actively to extend the scope of public-health work. In 1909, Lillian Wald drew Metropolitan Life Insurance into public-health nursing. Eager to preserve their subscribers from costly disability or premature death, MLI became an important corporate sponsor of public-health projects. By 1921 it had 1,222 centers, was affiliated with 887 visiting nurses' associations, and employed 338 of its own nurses to work exclusively with MLI clients. Other nurses worked to reshape their services into the emerging mold of preventive care. Mary Sewall Gardner's approach in Providence, Rhode Island, an early example, became a model for many other agencies. Established in 1900, the district nursing agency had been a philanthropic project to serve the sick and "worthy" poor. Gardner took over in 1905 and reorganized the service along the broader lines of the public-health perspective. She divided the city into districts and added systematic case-finding, prenatal instruction, and child welfare programs to the traditional work of bedside care. Gardner also expanded the agency's sphere of activity beyond the usual beneficiaries. Defining the whole city as part of the constituency for public-health services, she actively sought paying clients. She hoped that eventually fees from wealthier clients could fund care to the poor, freeing the agency from dependence on philanthropic or municipal funding. Meanwhile, private contributions, insurance fees, and public appropriations kept the agency going. Described in her manual *Public Health Nursing*, Gardner's citywide plan influenced visiting nurses' associations elsewhere and indicated the sweeping goals of public-health reformers.[5]

The continuing expansion of public health provided a rich field for nurses' endeavors. While the coming of the war checked much Progressive reform, it gave the public-health message a new urgency. Military induction physicals exempted thousands of young men from service on medical

grounds. The rejection rate probably reflected rising expectations of health, rather than any absolute decline in the fitness
of Americans. With advances in diagnosis and treatment,
military physicians applied more exacting standards and
screening to potential recruits. But whatever the explanation,
"the amazing discovery . . . that 29% of our young men were
physically unfit for military duty" made Americans especially
receptive to public-health initiatives.[6]

Programs that had been established before the war grew
rapidly with infusions of new funds in the wake of the war. In
1912, a gift from Henry Street philanthropists (arranged by
the ubiquitous Wald) had funded rural public-health programs
under the direction of the Red Cross. The plan provided
money for administrative and supervisory expenses in rural
agencies if local people could cover the nurse's salary. The
service grew slowly before the war, as reformers focused on
the crowded living conditions and immigrant populations of
the cities. In 1915, the Red Cross's Town and Country Service
employed only forty or fifty nurses. The findings of World
War I physicals modified this urban emphasis, turning more
public health efforts toward rural services. The sentimental
image of healthy country life yielded to a new perception of
rural decline. The high rejection rate of men from rural areas
led observers to conclude that "the country lad is less enduring, more prone to preventable physical disability, than his
city brothers." Epidemiological studies confirmed this: tuberculosis death rates were higher in many rural areas than in
urban centers, and typhoid fever, under control in the cities,
still presented a serious hazard to rural communities. The new
concern for rural health was reflected in the reorganization and
expansion of the Red Cross service. By 1921, 1,300 nurses
worked in small towns and rural areas under this program.[7]

The war also spurred efforts to confront venereal disease.
Defying public protests, the military had set into motion the
first large-scale campaign to educate soldiers about sexually
transmitted disease and to instruct them in prophylaxis. As
Salvarsan came into use and sexual mores became somewhat

more permissive, treatment of venereal disease became a technological and social possibility. The work presented a formidable challenge to public-health nurses. Patients were reluctant to identify themselves or their contacts, and many doctors resisted efforts to include screening for venereal disease in their routine examinations. The suppressed symptoms of syphilis made it difficult to diagnose, and, once brought to treatment, patients often defected before the end of the unpleasant, long, and unreliable regimen used in the 1920s. Gonorrhea had more marked symptoms, but before the discovery of penicillin in the 1940s, it too was difficult to control. One public-health manual estimated an infection rate of 40 to 60 percent for the whole male population. This statistic seems unreliably high, but, whatever its accuracy, it does convey the postwar concern with venereal disease. As uneasy civilians prepared for returning soldiers, the government followed military venereal disease programs with the Chamberlain-Kahn Act of 1918, providing money for state-administered programs of case-finding and treatment.[8]

Finally, the maternity and infant-care programs of the Sheppard-Towner Act became the backbone of public-health efforts in the 1920s. Sheppard-Towner was carried through Congress in the wake of women's suffrage, passed in 1921 after vigorous lobbying by feminist and Progressive reformers. The product of these reform energies, Sheppard-Towner also benefited from the public concern generated by the World War I findings. Supporters of the bill reminded their audiences of the disturbing results of the physicals and pointed out that healthy children would grow into healthy adults, the mothers and soldiers of the next generation. The legislation made federal funding available to states that could raise matching funds. By the end of the decade, forty-five states had organized prenatal and infant-care programs. The pregnant woman and her children presented sweeping opportunities for public-health nurses, and the financial and organizational structure of Sheppard-Towner facilitated the work. The large potential constituency of maternity and infancy programs presented a ready-made audience for the public-health message. The focus on child-raising gave public-health nurses access to whole families, extending the possibilities for casefinding and health education. Not surprisingly, maternal and infant welfare programs were the most common activities of public-health nursing agencies throughout the 1920s and 1930s.[9]

With this heightened attention to preventive care, publichealth nurses looked toward a promising future. The increased use of tax funding for public-health work offered a measure of its growing legitimacy. As the methods and messages of preventive medicine took hold, state and federal appropriations steadily assumed a larger role in public-health budgets. Agencies continued to draw on traditional philanthropic sources, to use Red Cross funding, and to derive income from insurance companies. But by the mid-1920s, only 25 percent ran on private funding alone, and nearly half of all public-health agencies were entirely supported by tax money. The numbers of public-health nurses had increased rapidly with the growing momentum of the preventive movement. In 1901, just 130 nurses had reported themselves as public-health nurses, a fraction of the nearly two thousand "trained nurses" listed in the 1900 census. By 1912, 3,000 nurses worked in public health, still a small segment of the 80,000 nurses in the 1910 count. A 1924 census of publichealth nurses documented a fivefold increase, enumerating 11,152 nurses. By 1926, nearly one-fifth of all nurses worked in public health.[10]

As preventive work expanded, a small but highly selfconscious group of nurses had begun to distinguish themselves from private-duty and hospital nurses. At the American Nurses' Association convention in 1912, 69 nurses gathered to establish the National Organization for Public Health Nursing (NOPHN), asserting their claim to a separate identity within nursing. For the first time, nurses in the visiting nurses' associations, anti-tuberculosis organizations, rural health agencies, and industrial dispensaries officially declared their common commitment to the broader public-health movement and symbolically joined their diverse efforts under the new label that Lillian Wald had suggested, "public-health nursing." Fittingly, Wald, who had done so much to create the institutions of public-health nursing, was named president. Nurse, educator, and reformer, she represented the mixture of professional ideology and broad social commitment that fueled nurses' participation in preventive care.[11]

The NOPHN provided a form and a structure for strengthening the links among widely scattered nurses engaged in diverse activities. After the convention, Ella Phillips Crandall, the newly elected secretary, traveled around the country to publicize the new organization, to observe different public-health activities, and to advise new endeavors. As an early historian of public-health nursing wrote, "It seemed as though, all at once, they were not alone, they had each and all become a great band with other workers." In language that recalled the ties between nineteenth-century reform and women's culture, Gardner celebrated "the feeling of sisterhood and the bond of a common purpose that bind all public health nurses together wherever their work may lie."[12]

The lofty rhetoric of reform provided a common ideology to inspire nurses in their daily labors. "A public health nurse is not an isolated unit trying to meet unique conditions in some particular locality," one manual explained. "She is . . . part of a large and important movement that is making itself felt all over the world." Confronting the setbacks and discouragements of local work, the nurse could take comfort in "a sense of belonging to something much bigger than herself, of having an important part in a great undertaking." This ideology cast public-health nurses in a newly self-conscious social role. "They believe in the dignity and value of their daily lives, knowing that they are part of a great constructive social force which must in the end correct much that is unbearable in our present social structure." A contributor to *Public Health Nursing* wrote: "There are great heights to be reached. There are mountains not yet in sight to be climbed."[13]

With the formation of the NOPHN, public-health nurses acknowledged their connections to reformers and to other nurses and simultaneously declared their independence from both groups. By uniting nurses across institutional boundaries, from settlement houses to factories, the NOPHN asserted its members' common interests and outlook *as nurses* in the public-health movement. NOPHN organizers claimed an autonomous role within preventive care, implicitly declaring their legitimate right to direct and organize the nursing activities related to public health. At the same time, by forming a separate association at the ANA convention, they put nursing leaders on notice that public-health work had its own agenda, one that went beyond the concerns represented by the existing professional associations. Both the ANA and the National League of Nursing Education (NLNE) were committed to the goal of professionalization, and both interpreted public service primarily in this context: a well-regulated and well-educated profession would best meet the needs of laypersons. The NOPHN turned from this internal concern with nursing as an occupation to seek a broader working alliance with public-health reformers, setting a self-conscious distance between itself and professional associations for nursing. Public-health nurses underlined their relationship to Progressive reform by opening membership to laypersons and actively soliciting lay involvement in the agencies. At the founding meeting, they emphasized that the NOPHN was to be an organization for public health *nursing*—a cooperative effort of professionals and laypersons committed to the movement, not an organization designed to represent nurses' specific professional interests.

However, public-health nurses did bring professional aspirations of their own to reform activity. The special opportunities and borrowed prestige of the public-health movement gave these nurses the reputation of an elite corps within nursing, an identity they protected with a jealous exclusiveness. Just as leaders in the ANA and the NLNE tried to raise educational standards to restrict access to nursing, NOPHN leaders struggled to limit entry to public health by creating a credential to separate public-health nurses from other nurses. As early as 1912, its founding year, the NOPHN was preparing that ground by devising postgraduate courses in public-health nursing. The organization consistently rejected attempts to incorporate training for public health into the hospital school curriculum, choosing instead to reserve it for a postgraduate specialization.[14]

The NOPHN never fully controlled access to the field, and, like ANA and NLNE investigations, its surveys repeatedly documented the gap between the standards they advocated and nurses' actual qualifications. Public health retained flexible hiring practices. It was a relatively new nursing specialty: indeed, few formal public-health nursing courses were available in the 1920s and 1930s. The NOPHN itself continued to recognize experience as an equivalent credential to coursework for all but the highest positions in public health. Perhaps more important, public-health nurses worked for many different institutions, from municipal health departments to nurse-run agencies to industrial clinics, not all of which were equally receptive to guidance from the NOPHN.[15]

Yet although public-health nurses fell short of the NOPHN's recommended standards, they stood well above most other nurses. By the measures of aspiring professionals, public-health nurses did constitute an elite. They had more education than their counterparts in private duty and on hospital staffs, and, on the average, they could claim more credentials than even supervisory or administrative nurses in hospitals. Many public-health nurses were recruited from the more prestigious schools of nursing in larger hospitals, another measure of stature within nursing. Women in public-health supervision and administration stood at the pinnacle of their occupation, boasting stronger educational backgrounds than any other group of nurses.[16]

Like other elite nurses, public-health nurses often used education as a code for class, and, like Progressive reformers, they often brought a strong strain of nativism to their visions of social amelioration. The appropriate expert, in the public-health and the Progressive perspective, was middle class, native-born, and white. Public-health agencies sought the "high type well educated nurse"; as one administrative nurse explained, "Public health nursing demands a young woman who has family background and ideals, so that almost unknowingly she inculcates." In many areas, foreign-born nurses were excluded because they lacked "the environment and training" of native-born Yankee Americans. Black women, generally underrepresented in nursing, were rarely found among public-health nurses. The exception was in the southern states, where racism reversed the argument used against foreign-born nurses. Especially in rural districts, public-health agencies used black nurses for their black clients with an alacrity that seemed to come more from white nurses' reluctance to cross color lines than from an enlightened appreciation for black colleagues. The "gospel of health" remained largely the ministry of the elect, a situation that would strongly influence public-health nurses' relationships to doctors, clients, and other nurses.[17]

Public-health nursing was colored by both nineteenth-century moral reform and the Progressive enthusiasm for technological solutions administered by experts. Nurses allied with the public-health movement used rhetoric that recalled the traditional conception of nursing as Christian service. One manual urged nurses to lead the great procession toward "the promised land of municipal health," and others called their teaching "the gospel of health" or the counsel of "right living." Public-health nurses infused their health education with the drama of moral struggle, and their fervor expressed itself even in the most mundane teaching devices. The *Maternity Handbook*, for example, purveyed its advice as "The Ten Commandments of Health," and a campaign in the schools to wean children from pernicious stimulants posed "the triumph of good over evil—milk versus coffee." Public-health nurses described their relationships with patients in terms that recalled the traditional private-duty nurse's sense of womanly duty and intimate involvement with patients; as a Red Cross campaign put it, they were the "mothers of the world."[18]

But the language of public health also reflected the growing professionalization of reform. Nurses sought a more scientific method, a rational approach to the goal of better health. Public health was too important to be left to amateurs, even if they were dutiful women: a new layer of experts interpreted preventive medicine and guided its applications. In its funding and philosophy, preventive care moved from its charitable origins and paternalistic ethos toward a view of health as a concern of the state, a way to ensure national security and productivity. The tension between these conflicting traditions lay at the core of public-health nursing in the 1920s and 1930s.

II. "NURSE, TEACHER, COUNSELOR, AND FRIEND"

Leaders in public-health nursing seized the chance to assert their special expertise in the uncharted and unclaimed territory of preventive medicine. The NOPHN's journal, *The Public Health Nurse* (later *Public Health Nursing*), portrayed nurses as the vanguard of the movement. In the 1920s and 1930s, public-health nurses published a number of manuals, didactic novels, and histories that both reflected and fostered the development of a distinctive nursing specialty. This literature reinterpreted nurses' province and responsibilities in the altered context of preventive care. Manuals emphasized health education as the special contribution of the public-health nurse, minimizing the traditional tasks of bedside nursing: "The nurse who tends the sick only, and teaches nothing and prevents nothing, is abortive in her work." Like other aspiring professionals, public-health nurses stressed the broad theoretical basis of their work. Experts in the "laws" of health, public-health nurses moved beyond the traditional service relationships of nursing to claim a newly autonomous role. They were teachers, "the indispensable carriers of the findings of the scientists and the laboratories to the people themselves."[19]

The organization of public health facilitated nurses' independence on the job. The work settings of public health removed nurses from direct medical control. Public-health nursing associations (PHNAs) were directed by nurses who worked with lay boards. Their funding came primarily from private sources; they were also called voluntary or nonofficial agencies. The PHNAs covered the widest variety of work, active in both traditional and preventive fields. They cared for sick patients in their homes, a service in constant demand. Working to promote preventive care, they also mounted maternity and infant programs, vaccination campaigns, casefinding and follow-up efforts. In state or municipal health departments, public-health nurses worked under nursing directors or health officers, who might be either laypersons or salaried doctors. These nurses usually did little or no bedside care, concentrating on contagious disease control, screening, and "health education," a label that could cover a multitude of services. Local boards of education often hired their own school nurses, who measured students' height and weight, administered eye examinations and dental inspections, indoctrinated their charges with "health habits," and segregated students with suspicious symptoms. Finally, a few factories and stores employed nurses to head their dispensaries. In these settings, nurses applied first aid, kept employee health records, ran screening and educational campaigns, and sometimes conducted plant inspections to make recommendations about safety on the job.

Under these novel conditions, nurses' authority was extended beyond the traditional bounds set by medical prerogatives. While public-health nurses formally worked under doctors' orders, physicians often supervised them from afar. Many nurses obtained standing orders, drawing up general protocols for treatment and getting the local medical society to approve them. Such orders gave nurses the license to work without direct supervision while remaining within the law that governed medical and nursing practice. Industrial nurses applied first aid and performed minor treatments without doctors. In the PHNAs, bedside nursing care could be covered by standing orders for one or two visits, after which the patient had to call a doctor. But even in this area, closest to traditional medical and nursing care, physicians' authority might be remote. As one public-health nurse explained, doctors might never see their patients in person; rather, agency nurses could report and receive orders over the telephone.[20]

In isolated settings, public-health nurses took on many of the prerogatives usually reserved for doctors. A male nurse described his work in a depression camp for homeless men. "You are often called upon here to do things that you are never called to do in other hospitals. . . . In the absence of the physician, you are called sometimes to render a decision which may seem beyond your ability—thus a nurse learns to stand on his own feet." Another account illustrates nurses' liberal interpretation of professional ethics in such settings. A supervisor told about her tour to nurses in a remote Arctic outpost. One of her nurses solicited her advice on how to treat a woman with a badly infected finger. Lancing such an infection was a surgical procedure, strictly a medical prerogative. "I was the supervisor on trial," she remembered. "Would I transgress the unwritten law of nursing and medical practice?" She performed the procedure, but never acknowledged overtly that a nurse might take on medical duties. "I was mean enough not to let Miss Tiber know that I had seen through her ruse. . . . We let it go like that." In collusions like this, nurses could maintain their commitment to traditional ethics while transgressing them when necessary. In situations where such "exceptions" were common, the nurse's authority was implicitly expanded. Rural nurses in particular noted the enforced autonomy of their isolated work setting.[21]

Nurses' new roles in case-finding and health supervision eluded the existing definitions of medical and nursing prerogatives, and doctors were slow to assert an active control over preventive medicine. In situations that called for "health education," the nurse enjoyed considerable freedom, offering advice on diet, home hygiene, and child care. Maternity and infant-care programs, important activities of public-health nurses in the 1920s and 1930s, were almost exclusively supervised by nurses. Public-health nurses sought out the pregnant women in their districts, enrolled them in "mothers' classes," and persuaded them to see a doctor. Expectant mothers were supposed to consult their physicians three times before delivery, but most agencies accepted patients who visited a doctor once. With the mother officially under medical supervision, the nursing program could proceed. Public-health nurses saw their patients often, instructing them on diet and monitoring their progress. By 1930, some public-health nurses were measuring blood pressure and doing urinalyses for pregnant women, referring them to doctors if something was amiss. Although the discreet nurse would merely report her data and not diagnose overtly, the whole screening arrangement tacitly relegated a diagnostic function to the nurse.

Often public-health organizations had only sporadic contact with local doctors, reinforcing the autonomy that individual nurses claimed on the job. In 1924, a small NOPHN survey of visiting nurses' associations showed that six of fourteen agencies had no doctors on their boards, especially striking since these agencies provided much bedside care. By 1934, sixteen of twenty-one public-health nursing associations reported some formal relationship with physicians, but only five of these boards or medical advisory committees met regularly. Similarly, another study of 132 nonofficial agencies found that only 84 had formal medical advisory boards, and most did not hold regular meetings. Slightly under half (61) had doctors on their boards. Two-thirds of the nursing agencies in the NOPHN survey claimed that their relationships with local physicians were "friendly," but the same agencies indicated that doctors did not use their services. Of the sixteen associations that responded, only six reported that "many" or "the majority" of doctors in the community referred patients to them. One estimated that about one-third of the local doctors called on the agency, while nine admitted that "few" physicians worked with them.[22]

As these statistics suggest, public-health nurses' relationships with physicians were frequently tense and strained. Many doctors viewed preventive work with indifference or outright hostility. In complaints moderated by the laws of professional loyalty, public-health nurses acknowledged their struggles with recalcitrant physicians; as one wrote, "In dealing with doctors. . . . a nurse will have an opportunity to use her powers of adaptability to the full." In an article that described the organization of a new midwife-supervision program, the author gratefully acknowledged the ready assistance of child hygiene nurses, visiting nurses, hospital administrators, and lay health officers, then noted: "The general cooperation of the medical profession has not been so easy to gain." A tuberculosis nurse reported, "Another problem, and often a grave problem, is to gain the undivided cooperation and approval of the county medical society." Driven beyond such careful phraseology, an exasperated rural nurse complained, "The average country physician reminds one of the famous Scot who said, 'Thank God! *I* am not open to conviction!' "[23]

Physicians opposed public-health work in defense of their own professional prerogatives. The lay movement threatened doctors' claims to the exclusive right to define the content and organization of medical care, to control related services, and to work without constraints from outsiders. In a debate over a well-baby clinic, one doctor admitted the need for these new preventive services, but argued that providing them should remain strictly a medical prerogative. "Lay propaganda, welfare conferences, and public health measures . . . are only accessory methods and means." Although physicians were slow to become involved actively in public-health work themselves, they still resisted laypersons' and nurses' efforts to organize medical services. At the NOPHN conference in 1924, one doctor took the podium to complain of "the aggressiveness of the public health nurse." A rural nurse observed, "Doctors are rather scornful of the encroachment of public health nurses and sanitarians into the medical field."[24]

The funding of public health was a source of bitter conflict between private physicians and public-health reformers. On the most mundane level, some physicians simply feared economic competition from free or low-priced services. In New Orleans, for example, the Child Welfare Association set off an explosive controversy when it proposed a free well-baby clinic. Private doctors panicked at the prospect of their paying clients flocking to the free service, and attempted to defeat the plan. The association's superintendent defended the clinic, denying the conflict of interest that physicians feared. Clients had to be persuaded to seek out care for well children, she asserted, and would not yet pay for the service even if they could afford it. On a more aggressive tack, she concluded by demanding, "Is there a danger of protecting the economic interests of the physician at the expense of the patients . . . ?"[25]

On a deeper level, public-health nurses and private doctors were divided by fundamentally different social visions. Many physicians clung to a paternalistic approach that nurses were discarding in favor of an environmental approach to reform. The private practitioners represented by the American Medical Association were social conservatives, believers in the virtues of the free market and the evils of state control. At work they were individualists, each building his own following of loyal patients, and they were ardent defenders of fee-for-service practice as the appropriate vehicle for the personal relationship between doctor and patient. Doctors had always provided a measure of free service too, and they repeatedly insisted that they were committed to serving anyone who needed care. But they wanted such services clearly defined as philanthropy and dispensed under the control of the medical profession.

One debate tellingly illustrates the sharp differences between public-health nurses and doctors. Protesting nurses' more liberal use of free services, one doctor warned against the pernicious moral effects of "offering [patients] for nothing things that they ought to pay for." Such profligacy opened the door to further ills. "Furnish [bedside nursing] free to all and see whom we have here! Our old friend State Medicine or

Socialized Medicine." In a crisp editorial, a public-health nurse replied that patients were demoralized by illness and worries about medical bills, not by free nursing services. She rejected the physician's individualism for the environmental perspective of public health. "Faulty conditions in our towns and cities are largely responsible for the illnesses of the poor. . . . 'Push while the family pulls' is a good visiting nurse slogan; and perhaps we can suggest another: 'Mend the road.' "[26]

Private doctors consistently resisted any public initiatives that appeared to threaten private medicine, either in practice or in principle. The 1934 NOPHN survey explored physicians' objections to public-health programs. The data revealed that medical resistance was strongest against tax-supported boards of education. School nurses attended students of all income levels, arousing doctors' fears of competition. School nursing programs, which were funded by local governments, were also a red flag to physicians set against state medicine. Doctors reacted more favorably to visiting nurses' associations, which served a predominantly poor clientele and often depended on private sources of funding.[27]

In journal articles and manuals, nurses discussed methods for managing difficult doctors. Prescriptive literature counseled nurses to avoid conflict by strictly observing professional ethics. Because public-health nurses often worked without the direct supervision of a doctor, they had to make special efforts to demonstrate their symbolic deference to medical authority. A school nurse warned others to tread carefully with hostile physicians, adhering rigidly to the codes of respect for medical prerogatives. "It is never wise to say 'adenoids' no matter how sure you are—merely 'nasal obstruction.' It may save endless difficulties with touchy physicians."[28] Others charged nurses to avoid open criticism of doctors, and to stress to their clients that they were working under the physician's invisible hand (even though he was seldom in evidence). Cultivating medical support in the community was one of the avowed goals of every public-health nursing association. Manuals repeatedly emphasized the importance of establishing formal relationships with local doctors through medical advisory committees.

But underlying this dutiful recitation of traditional nursing ethics was a certain ambivalence about the physician's place in public health. One comment betrayed its author's skepticism about the average run of doctors. Reminding nurses of their duty to be tolerant and to reserve judgment of medical superiors, she wrote, "An open mind will often discover ability where it is least expected." Although manuals and journal articles urged closer working relationships with doctors, in practice public-health nurses seemed reluctant to admit physicians to the governing boards of the agencies. In one survey, the NOPHN asked public-health nursing associations if they thought doctors should be on the boards. Of 132 agencies, only 43 found them useful, 14 opposed the idea outright, and, in the eloquent silence of professional etiquette, 75 voiced no opinion. Nurses supported their lay boards, affirming the public-health movement's commitment to lay involvement and at the same time giving themselves a buffer against medical interference.[29]

Doctors' absence from public health created opportunities for nurses to step into the gap as the ranking experts. Conscious of the expanded scope of nursing in public health, some set forth an explicit rationale to defend their autonomy. In a notable departure from the more common indirection, public-health nurses sometimes baldly asserted that they were the legitimate authorities in preventive care. A manual on school nursing openly challenged doctors' traditional control. "The physician, because of his medical proficiency, is nominally in charge of the situation, but is he really? The nurse . . . knows the principal, the teachers, the families of her children. The physician does not. Practically, then, the nurse really is in the best position to 'run the show.' " More often, nurses struggled to maintain their authority by bolstering their positions in the organizational structure of public health. The manuals strongly recommended nurse-controlled agencies.

Gardner advised municipal health departments to maintain separate divisions of nursing with their own budgets and nurse-administrators. "Entirely apart from the efficiency of work which is almost invariably increased by nurse directorship, the psychological effect on a staff of the leadership of a member of the same profession is far-reaching." Another manual declared, "It is through the supervision of public health nurses by public health nurses that efficient . . . nursing services will be developed."[30]

Faced with an unreliable medical profession, nurses and reformers recognized that the survival of their work depended on their ability to mobilize lay support. Their mission was to spread the gospel of health, to educate and inspire laypersons to demand the benefits of preventive medicine. "When the desire cometh, it is a tree of life," the NOPHN motto counseled, and nurses worked hard to plant and cultivate it.

Laypersons often dragged their feet down the road to "right living," skeptical of the millennial promises of preventive medicine and loath to seek out medical guidance except in sickness. School nurses promoted toothbrushes, balanced diets, and tonsillectomies to doubtful audiences. Parents resented school nurses' inspections of their children and sometimes refused to follow up on their findings. In prenatal and infant care, public-health nurses struggled to assert new standards and practices against long-established lay traditions. Black and immigrant women often refused the care of male doctors, clinging to seasoned midwives. Everywhere, pregnant women and new mothers depended on the lore of their female friends and relatives, and turned only reluctantly from these networks to self-proclaimed experts in nursing and medicine.

Nurses' efforts to promote a new view of health revealed the dual potential of the movement itself. On the one hand, public-health work expressed a genuinely democratic impulse: nurses sought to bring the benefits of scientific medicine to people who were largely neglected by private practitioners. Highly conscious of the intimidating aura of medicine, they worked to win their patients' trust and to speak in a language that laypersons could understand. Often they encouraged traditions of self-help and mutual aid. At its best, public health embodied a commitment to make medicine both accessible and accountable.

On the other hand, the broader definition of health also led to a kind of medical imperialism. By bringing virtually every aspect of human activity under the rubric of health, public-health ideology provided a justification for greatly expanded medical intervention: "the mere absence of disease" did not deter experts bent on providing for "the individual's needs, his welfare, efficiency, and happiness."[31] Welded to the elitism underlying Progressive reform and to the public-health nurse's exalted self-image, this diffuse definition of health could become the instrument for the imposition of dominant values. The goal of "right living" gave free rein to class, ethnic, and racial prejudices. Good health could become a code for middle-class standards and practices, and, like other types of reform, public health could become a vehicle for social control.

The redefinition of health also reached across class lines to work a far-reaching cultural transformation. Alongside its traditions of self-help, public health prepared the way for the extension of medical expertise into more and more areas of life. Ivan Illich has criticized the "creation of dependence" that has followed medical expansion. As experts claim control over sickness and health, laypersons lose confidence in traditional means of coping. The tyranny of "expert opinion" overrides personal judgment and older familial or community resources. If public-health reformers began by challenging the limits of fee-for-service practice, they ended, not by transforming medicine, but by extending its scope and producing new consumers for it.[32]

Eager to claim their own places as experts, public-health nurses were not immune from the prejudices of professional ideology. At times, they aggressively promoted middle-class respectability with their patients. Closely linked to settlement-house work, public-health reform was colored by both the Progressive faith in assimilation and its unself-conscious chauvinism. Nurses portrayed domestic and personal hygiene as "American," and used individuals' "health habits" as a measure of their assimilation. Their accounts of work in immigrant neighborhoods convey both the optimism of Progressive reform and the lingering association of immigrants with dirt and contagion. Describing a campaign against lice, one public-health nurse concluded, "Aside from handling the health problem we believe that if we have created a desire for a clean head and a clean body we have taken one long step toward 'Americanizing' the people with whom we are working." In another piece, "Making Billy Safe for Democracy," a nurse teaches an immigrant mother how to care for a son, who has diphtheria, at home. A dental-care program was described under the grandiose title "Making Better Americans." The aggressive mood of "100% Americanism" showed in another nurse's teaching device for her Native American and Spanish-speaking students in New Mexico. For each health habit acquired, the child got to add one pane of colored tissue paper to the "Magic Window." When the panes were filled in, the nurse would award the central panel, a rendition of a boy and girl in military caps carrying the flag. As the nurse explained, this represented "the wonderful picture of what they themselves would become—good Americans—by the daily practising of health habits."[33]

Prescriptions for child-raising clearly indicated the middle-class ideals that informed nurses' notions of right living, for here too proper child care was overtly equated with "American" habits. A nurse from Connecticut noted with satisfaction, "Many an Italian and Polish youngster has been transformed in the twinkling of an eye into a little American citizen by a mere change of clothing." Regularity, discipline, and early independence were the goals of child care. Nurses inspected the households in their districts and approved clean, quiet, uncluttered, and well-organized quarters. Guided by her public-health nurse, one enterprising young mother divided her day into fifteen-minute periods, filling these slots with different jobs. The *Maternity Handbook* advised the mother to keep daily records, noting the child's eating habits, stools, sun baths, and behavior. For efficient child care, nurses recommended early toilet training, sleeping alone, and the firm discipline of schedules.[34]

Public-health nurses were undoubtedly influenced by the nativism of the 1920s and the ingrained prejudices of their class, reinforced by their claim to professional expertise. Still, in the 1920s and 1930s, these attitudes were held in check by the precarious position of public health. Traditional medical and nursing practice operated with the advantages of well-established networks of referrals and in the context of a clear lay demand for services. Operating without strong medical support, nurses had to work actively to win the loyalty and patronage of laypersons. Offering new and unfamiliar services, they also had to create a demand for public health. As one nurse noted, "Almost anyone could sell Fords or South Florida real estate, or something that people really wanted. But to sell positive health . . . requires good salesmanship indeed."[35] Under these circumstances, nurses were forced to temper their standards with tolerance of other ways.

More positively, the public-health movement itself contained models and values that countered nurses' class and professional predilections. Retaining their roots in the settlement-house movement, public-health nurses tried to reconcile the goal of assimilation with a respect for ethnic diversity. Manuals repeatedly cautioned nurses to adapt their teaching to immigrants' cultural traditions and not to assume that their own ways were best. Like settlement-house efforts to preserve ethnic crafts even as the goal of assimilation undermined the ways of life that had supported them, public-health nurses' adaptations were sometimes superficial. One frequently used exemplar of flexibility suggests the level at which compromise came most easily: prescriptive literature encouraged nurses to accommodate rural or immigrant customs and preferences in advice on healthy diets.[36]

Other examples, though, showed nurses making larger compromises and learning from their clients. In "Infant Feeding Trials in the Mountains," one nurse offered a thoughtful cautionary tale. "With the ardor of a newcomer," she remembered, she had tried to get rural mothers and babies on the regular feeding schedules and diet approved in the child welfare literature. But the mountain families had no clocks, thus thwarting her best efforts to apply middle-class discipline. In pursuit of the goal of early independence, she encouraged mothers to wean their babies earlier. The first demonstration ended in near disaster, for, once weaned, the baby "almost faded out of sight." The nurse recognized belatedly that, in this setting, children needed prolonged breast-feeding, for the fresh vegetables and easily digestible foods of a good infant diet were not available. Throughout the 1920s and 1930s, public-health nurses displayed a similar adaptability and openness to local customs in their relationships with midwives. Unlike most physicians, nurses accepted lay midwives and simply armed them with better techniques. Prescriptive literature emphasized the value of open-mindedness, and public-health nurses prided themselves on their highly personal and flexible approach to patients. "We are attempting to find out what it is that the patient wants from the nurse and what, because of his individual capabilities and situation, he will be able to use. It is *his* situation, *his* life."[37]

Common propaganda techniques indicated nurses' efforts to meet potential clients on their own ground. Drawing contrasts between themselves and their more aloof medical colleagues, nurses struggled to insert health information into popular culture. After World War I, Red Cross nurses traveled with the Chautauqua vaudeville entertainers to spread their message, regaling crowds with stories of their war experiences and exhorting them to hire county nurses. *Public Health Nursing* publicized and supported the National Health Organization's 1923 campaign to promote preventive consultations with the slogan "Have a health examination on your birthday!" In their districts, nurses recruited pregnant women for prenatal classes and held "mothercraft" meetings to prepare young girls for their maternal destinies. Publicity campaigns used department store window displays, posters, newspaper ads, and local radio broadcasts. School nursing programs persuaded children with didactic stories and plays, featuring the Child Health Organization's health fairy and her sidekick "Cho Cho, the Health Clown." Nurses turned boosterism to their own purposes by sponsoring activities like the national Chamber of Commerce competition for the healthiest city. "Syracuse wishes you well," one magnanimous winner proclaimed. Children paraded through town costumed as "the vegetable battalion." Pageants and live demonstrations provided other media for publicizing public health. Such techniques suggested the limits of public-health reformers' challenges to mainstream medicine, for they used the developing methods of advertising to create new medical consumers. But within the limits of that structure, they made information about health more accessible and encouraged clients of health services to become better informed.[38]

Prescriptive literature stressed personal, respectful relationships with patients as the key to successful public-health work. Aware of their uncertain reception, nurses counseled ingenuity and tact in approaching the patient at home. A didactic story illustrated the ideal methods. In advising a reluctant Italian family, the nurse "showed no spirit of officiousness. . . . Like a ray of sunshine she came, and the place began to bloom. . . . She radiated good health. . . . She treated Mrs. Annuzzo as a personal friend." A public-health manual cited another exemplary case history: "Her method was indirect. . . . By an adroit question or two she drew out the difficulties presented by both children, all the time listening and giving the mother time to pour out all her troubles. At appropriate moments she offered suggestions and new ideas, making the procedures sound attractive and possible." Over and over, case histories in *PHN* demonstrated the subtle methods of tactful intervention. In one didactic story, a young nurse drives over rugged roads to reach a case of suspected meningitis. She discovers that this patient has already been hospitalized, but, ever alert for opportunities to teach health, she strikes up a conversation with a pregnant bystander. Before her unsuspecting victim can resist, the nurse has persuaded her to get prenatal care, collected a urine specimen, and arranged a vaccination for her toddler.[39]

The emphasis on an individual approach to laypersons was more than rhetorical: by the mid-1920s, it had led to a restructuring of the agencies, as public-health nurses reversed the specialization that had begun to divide care among a number of nurses. The specialized service was a legacy of public health's early history: as lay groups like tuberculosis or child welfare associations promoted those services, health departments or nursing associations had added staff nurses to cover one kind of patient. Manuals criticized this division of labor, recommending instead the citywide plan of organization, which assigned nurses to all the households in a district. Rather than visiting all the patients with tuberculosis in her city, or supervising all the young children, the nurse would care for the different needs of the people in her district. This arrangement gave variety and interest to the work and allowed considerable scope for nursing intervention. For example, the nurse might enter a home to answer the family's call for bedside nursing of a child with pneumonia. Once inside, she could observe the whole family's situation and offer hints on child-raising, arrange corrective surgery for a child with a twisted back, have a coughing adult tested for tuberculosis. By 1934, all of the nursing agencies in the NOPHN survey had returned to the generalized service. "The public health nurse is the family health worker," declared Lillian Wald.[40]

The public-health nurse's relationship to her patient drew on both the older values of women's culture and the newer aspirations of professional ideology. Public-health nurses affirmed the special intimacy of their work in terms that recalled the traditional private-duty nurse's relationships. "I have found that I have a more personal feeling toward my patients, which I never could have obtained in the hospital

surroundings," one student wrote. Another nurse fondly remembered her eighteen years in one Brooklyn district; long
association had drawn her into the life of the Italian neighborhood. Lillian Wald's memoirs evoked the rich community life
of settlement-house workers. A 1930s public-health nurse
remembered the satisfaction of following her patients over the
years.[41]

Public-health districts substituted for the social networks
that some private-duty nurses had enjoyed, and many public-
health nurses echoed the older rhetoric of womanly service.
"You have prepared yourselves to be trained foster mothers in
your district," one superintendent told her fledgling public-
health nurses. "Just as the mother is alive *to* and interested *in* all
the needs—physical, mental, spiritual—of her child, just so
your people will recognize in you a sympathy and human
interest." Another wrote, "Perhaps the old district patient . . .
defined a nurse when she said . . . 'She's been a mother to me,
that visiting nurse has, a real mother.' "[42]

Exchanging wealthy patients for a clientele in more modest circumstances, public-health nurses could recover some of
the intimacy of private duty without relinquishing their control as workers. One nurse's story illustrated the psychological and social gains of treating poorer patients. After leaving a
job in a New York City slum neighborhood for a less hectic
job in the suburbs, she developed a severe facial paralysis. "In
the new position the nurse had lost all her sense of security and
importance. Her patients belonged, for the most part, to a
class of considerable wealth and assured social position."
Their businesslike attitude and resistance to her advice left the
nurse feeling "snubbed, inferior, and crushed." She left for a
new job in an isolated rural district "with a group of people
who look up to her and respect her intelligence, and who again
contribute to her sense of well-being and happiness in her
work." In the 1920s, 88 percent of public-health nurses had
worked in private duty, and some left their wealthy patients
with open relief. As one wrote, "There is greater satisfaction
in doing for these poor unfortunates than in catering to pa-

tients who have lived lives of pampered luxury." Another
nurse noted, "You meet a class of people who need your care
and advice. . . . One is more appreciated."[43]

While public-health nurses might regain some of the old
satisfactions of private duty, their new setting and altered
status fundamentally reshaped their relationships with patients. For traditional private-duty nurses, personal ties with
patients were ends in themselves; for public-health nurses,
they were methods aimed towards larger goals. Public-health
nurses saw their intimacy with patients more instrumentally,
as a means to convert the doubtful to the gospel of health. As
one wrote, "Our success does not count in the huge piles of
figures we may turn in . . . but very much more . . . where we
have just loved people into right living." The manuals praised
close relationships with patients as an efficacious method; a
pragmatic approach began to replace the social and religious
values of traditional women's culture.

> It is usually taught in hospitals that a nurse should not
> intrude her own joys and sorrows upon her patients. For
> the public health nurse such advice requires modification.
> Her influence lies in her power to gain the confidence and
> affection of her patients. And who confides in or grows
> fond of an impersonal being who gives nothing of herself
> in return?

Even as public-health nurses affirmed their close relationships
with patients, they revealed a growing commitment to the
image of the nurse as expert. In a phrase that aptly rendered
this blend of traditional and professional ideology, the
NOPHN manual named the public-health worker "nurse,
teacher, counselor, and friend."[44]

Joining the values of the older tradition to newer efforts
for uniform professional standards, public-health nurses
worked to develop a formula that would reliably produce the
best of the old relationships between nurse and patient. Both
NOPHN surveys centered on evaluating public-health pro-

grams. In the 1924 study, the committee used questionnaires, interviews, and observation of the work to assess agencies. By 1934, the NOPHN had abandoned this rather impressionistic method for a detailed quantitative system of evaluation. In this search for an objective, "scientific" basis for nursing methods, public-health nursing leaders revealed their kinship with the educational reformers in the American Nurses' Association and the National League of Nursing Education.[45]

Even in the 1920s, worried observers noted the contradiction embedded in the public-health nursing ideology, the tension between traditional values and the growing professionalization of nursing and social service. One public-health leader conveyed the early spirit of the movement even as she warned:

> The professional, the scientific, the purely business side of her work must never overshadow the warm, human side; she must still be not only a teacher, but a friend, so that those who are to benefit by her teaching and her care will say, not "There goes our public health teacher,"— but "There goes Our Nurse."[46]

As this author recognized, the 1920s and 1930s was a time of a delicate balance that could not endure. Doctors' absence was critical: the marginality of public health and its distance from mainstream medicine had opened up an unprecedented opportunity for nurses. But the successes of public health in the 1920s and 1930s undermined its special character in the 1940s and 1950s. As public health became more acceptable, it was absorbed into the institutions and, to a large degree, into the philosophy of mainstream curative medicine. With the reorganization of public health, the nurse would lose much of her old autonomy, to return to a subordinate position in a rationalized and bureaucratic system of delivery. The special nurse-patient relationship of public health would be modified and diluted by the interposition of institutional care and the revival of specialization. And, finally, public-health nurses would feel the consequences of their own limits, for their perspective and self-organization could withstand neither the power of medical dominance nor the pull of professional ideology.

III. "EVERY NURSE A PUBLIC HEALTH NURSE"

By the 1930s, public health had scored resounding successes. Although Sheppard-Towner was defeated in 1929 by the American Medical Association, private medicine was steadily undergoing modification from forces both within and without the profession. The Committee on the Costs of Medical Care implicitly challenged the conservative control of the AMA. Established in 1926, the group set itself to investigate soaring costs and to estimate national medical needs. Gathering again at the 1927 meeting of the AMA, the Committee grew to fifty or sixty people, including physicians, nurses, hospital administrators, and concerned laypersons. The majority report of their 1932 national survey, *Medical Care for the American People*, returned again and again to the theme of preventive medicine and urged tax support for comprehensive public-health services. The routed AMA sponsored a minority report, signed by 17 of the 25 physicians on the committee; their dissent took the classic AMA position of opposing any shift from private fee-for-service practice. But other observers supported the development of health care in new directions, declaring that the United States needed forty to sixty thousand public health nurses, a considerable increase over the 24,000 listed in the 1930 public-health census. In 1937, mavericks within the medical profession protested AMA policies, forming the more socially conscious Committee of 430. During the depression and World War II, public health was a prominent concern in national planning, and state and federal funding grew. Relief programs recognized the medical needs of the indigent. The Social Security Act of 1935 provided a long-term basis for offering tax support to the blind, the disabled, and the elderly. World War II, like World War I, led to centralization of medical services in support of the military, and this time servicemen's families shared the benefits in a broad program of maternity and infant care.[47]

But as public-health services reorganized and expanded, nurses lost their autonomy and their distinctive identity along with their marginal status. Changing patterns of funding displaced the voluntary agencies that nurses had administered and controlled. Increasing specialization among public-health agencies disrupted the old ideal of generalized service. Within agencies, a new division of labor further revised the individual nurse-patient relationship of the 1920s.

As the depression spread, *Public Health Nursing* began to report losses of funding and personnel in the agencies, and the optimism of the 1920s yielded to a new, sober tone. Private contributions and income from patients' fees evaporated as the economy contracted, and the number of unemployed public-health nurses grew steadily. The NOPHN job registry swelled with nurses looking for work: in 1931 and 1932, the list lengthened to over a thousand names. *PHN* noted that inactive married and retired nurses were returning to the field as the depression cut into family incomes. Some nurses lost their jobs as nursing staffs shrank. In 1932, for example, 25 percent of the agencies in one study had cut nurses from their staffs, while only 9 percent reported any new positions; overall, the agencies lost 263 jobs. In 1929, the NOPHN had registered 836 jobs; in 1932, they listed only 364, and, of these, 83 were never funded. Meanwhile, case loads increased at an alarming rate as more and more people, unable to afford private-duty or hospital care, sought public-health nursing services.[48]

A number of depression programs provided funding for the struggling agencies. In 1931, the Federal and State Emergency Relief Administrations (FERA and SERA) began to set up nursing and medical programs for people on relief, and hired nurses on relief to work in them. The Civil Works Administration hired about six thousand nurses for short stints in a year-long program. Under the later Works Progress

Administration, another six thousand nurses were placed in local public-health projects for temporary employment. Some of this funding supported the increasing numbers of home visits for bedside nursing. Other state and federal programs underwrote dental care, immunization campaigns, nursery schools for children on relief, "home hygiene" and nutrition counseling, or the organization of new rural agencies.[49]

The NOPHN, fearing the effects of broader state involvement in the agencies, viewed the new funding with some apprehension. PHN warned that "constant care needs to be exercised to see that the emergency program supplements, but does not take the place of existing health programs, and to resist the temptation to hand over the established health programs to the emergency relief administration just because it has, at the moment, more funds." Throughout the depression, the NOPHN reminded its nurse and lay membership that public health was a specialized field, and urged careful selection of nurses on the projects; PHN pleaded, "Not Just Any Nurse, Please!" In the FERA projects, planners did agree to hire experienced or specially trained public health nurses first, but most of the nurses employed in the programs came straight from hospitals or private duty. Although most of the depression jobs lasted only a few months, the widespread participation of ordinary nurses probably blurred the distinctive identity of public-health nursing among nurses themselves and in their communities.[50]

The expanding public funding of the 1930s and 1940s altered the organization and the character of public-health nursing. Many of the services of the short-lived New Deal projects made their way into the 1935 Social Security Act, which extended existing funding for maternal and child welfare programs, initiated more rural public-health work, and offered some support to blind, disabled, and elderly citizens. But government funding tipped public-health nursing away from nonofficial agencies towards health departments and boards of education. Hit hard by the decline in private contributions and the dwindling numbers of paying patients, many of the voluntary agencies sought affiliations with the better-funded official agencies. In 1931, almost 40 percent of all public-health nurses had worked in the voluntary agencies; by 1938, these programs claimed only 25 percent of public-health nurses. Excluded from most of the new funding, the voluntary agencies never recovered from the depression. Between 1933 and 1948, the private agencies lost 23 percent of their nurses; during the same period, the staffs of health departments doubled, and boards of education hired fifty percent more school nurses.[51]

Administered by nurses and lay boards, the voluntary agencies had offered the most favorable environment of all the public health settings, fostering nursing initiative in the 1920s. Public-health nurses in these programs had the authority to plan and direct their own programs. Most of the staples of public-health work—tuberculosis case-finding and home care, prenatal and infant care, and school nursing—had been established through the experiments of private agencies. To many nurses, the work of the PHNAs represented the reform spirit of those years. One article pleaded for new methods of financing to preserve "the gadfly of the official agency," warning that "its absence in a community would leave untouched springs of spiritual life on which we are accustomed to rely to feed a social conscience, and which seem to be most readily released by the voluntary service and the attitude of mind developed by it."[52]

By the late 1930s, rationalization had overtaken public-health nursing. The generalized service gave way. Under new plans for coordinated community services, health departments and boards of education took over most preventive and educational work, relegating bedside nursing to private agencies. As all the agencies struggled to meet new demands for both preventive and bedside nursing services, the individual approach disappeared. Scrutinizing their services with a new eye for "efficiency," many agencies cut out the expensive and time-consuming tradition of home visiting. Visiting nurses' associations still cared for sick patients at home, but the work of health supervision moved to clinics and impersonal teaching conferences.[53]

The growing dominance of hospitals in the war and postwar years further altered public-health organization. During the 1940s, hospital out-patient clinics or social service departments assumed much of the work formerly done in agencies. Public-health nurses ran clinics and helped coordinate discharge and follow-up for hospital patients. While official agencies grew and voluntary agencies held on, the center of public health work had shifted to hospitals. By the late 1940s, *Public Health Nursing* referred to hospitals as "community health centers," and one doctor declared, "Rapidly the difference between public health and clinical nursing is becoming as difficult to distinguish as the imaginary line between preventive and curative medicine."[54]

In this institutional setting, new functions encroached on the nurse's relationship with her patient. Delivering out-patient services, public-health nurses functioned mostly as administrators, instructing hospital nurses about community social services and referring patients to them; as "liaison nurses," they had little direct contact with patients. In clinics, nurses saw many patients a day, but the hospital's tight schedules and uncongenial atmosphere constrained the old intimacy of home visiting. Working in hospitals, nurses lost some of the independence of public-health work to return to the traditional role of assisting doctors. Finally, the increased coordination of public-health agencies and hospitals reinforced the growing specialization of public-health nursing. Clinics and community referral services began to mimic the hospital's bureaucratic management and division of labor.

Some nurses protested the loss of public-health nursing's old identity and individuality. The impersonal approach of the clinics offended public-health veterans. "The 'case-hardened' attitude unfortunately so often still encountered among hospital personnel also carries over into clinics, obviously standing in the way of helping patients to make the fullest . . . use of the services available," one nurse wrote. The physician in charge of a venereal disease clinic reported that patients often disappeared before completing treatment, and he contrasted these dismal results with the successes of the visiting nurses. "You who meet the patient in his home have the advantage. . . . You meet the individual case, you convert the doubting, the hesitant, the weak or irresponsible, the uncomprehending." In another venereal disease clinic, a public-health nurse complained, "It was impossible to have a personal talk with each patient on account of the lack of time, space and personnel." Evaluating a tuberculosis clinic, another nurse severely criticized the routine and superficial interviewing that had replaced the close nurse-patient relationship of home visiting.[55]

Wartime demands and shortages of public-health nurses also pressed agencies toward greater division of labor. For the first time, discussions of auxiliary nursing services became a prominent feature of *PHN*. The agencies increased their use of volunteers, added part-time nurses who had no experience or training in public health, and began to hire practical nurses in public-health programs. A 1944 survey of 584 agencies showed that three-quarters had hired extra workers who were not trained in public health; one-quarter hired inactive graduate nurses and one-half used non-nurses. The journal published favorable reports of efficiency studies and urged agencies to reallocate their work. Like hospital rationalization, the resulting reorganization divided the tasks of the agency among several workers and created a new place for auxiliaries. In one official agency, clerical workers replaced twenty nurses, and graduate nurses took over clinic work that had been done by experienced public-health nurses. In the school nursing program, the public-health nurses trained teachers to carry out most of the inspection and health education.[56]

On the job, some public-health nurses resisted the trend toward division of labor, and the voluntary agencies defended the craft tradition of the early years. In 1948, for example, one survey found that only 8 percent of these associations used auxiliary nursing services, compared to 10 to 20 percent of the county health departments and 25 percent of municipal and state health departments. Workers who nursed for hire without a hospital school diploma had long been a presence in the ranks of the nursing workforce, and trained nurses often resented them as competitors who might undermine their wages and claims to special skill. After World War II, the so-called practical nurses began to claim new legitimacy with hospital administrators, physicians, and many nursing leaders. In the immediate postwar years, one- to two-year training courses stamped the practical nurse with a firmer identity, and state licensing followed in the 1950s (see Chapter 5). Like many other nurses, though, public-health nurses often resisted the use of an auxiliary worker who seemed to tread so close to nurses' traditional turf. In public-health agencies where practicals were introduced, nurses sometimes struggled to limit their responsibilities. One Boston supervisor admonished nurses for restricting auxiliary workers to "unnecessarily menial tasks" and belittling their work. In most agencies, practicals were banned from activities that involved health education, the traditional province of the public-health nurse.[57]

While practicals, aides, and clerks began to share the public-health nurse's routine tasks, other workers threatened the nurse's prerogatives in teaching and social services. Such new experts as nutritionists, physical therapists, and social workers all claimed special roles in public-health work. In the 1920s and 1930s, a few references in *PHN* had indicated the presence and growing professionalization of social workers. A psychiatric social worker implicitly staked out her own area of expertise, warning that nurses were "innocently harmful" in their unscientific approach to mental problems. Calling for a "professional" approach to social service, she criticized the highly individual approach prized in the public-health nursing manuals. "One hears the charge of social workers against nurses that they are sentimental, ruled by emotion, quick to act without knowing the whole situation." By the 1940s, social workers were edging nurses out of these roles altogether. "The public health nurse is not a trained social worker and the claim of nurses to dominate in this field has worked serious harm in certain communities," one public-health reformer noted severely in 1946. As social workers took jobs in public-health agencies, the division of labor was outlined. "The special contribution of the social worker lies in the area of handling complicated social and emotional problems. The special contribution of the nurse lies in the area of public health education." The nurse had formerly made her own decisions about her charges' special emotional or financial needs, and acted on those decisions herself. With the intervention of trained social workers, her responsibility was reduced to making appropriate referrals.[58]

Nurses and social workers clashed as public-health nurses struggled to defend their traditional role of "nurse, teacher, counselor, and friend" against the new division of labor. The two groups fought over the ambiguous boundaries of health education and social service. "In certain areas both nurses and social workers complain that the other encroaches upon her field," one social worker acknowledged. In a letter headed "Nurses and (or Versus) Social Workers," a nurse corroborated, "All too frequently there is friction between the social workers and the nurses in a community when they don't know what group does what for whom." An outraged nurse protested social workers' claim on psychiatric and social services, arguing that these were traditional and legitimate public-health nursing functions. Her criticism of social workers' patronizing airs reveals nurses' insecurity about these new experts. "We have had too much of this and I do not believe that there will ever be a healthy relationship between two professional groups when one insists upon assuming the role of teacher with superior knowledge."[59]

Other public-health nurses began to move toward a pragmatic acceptance of rationalization. Nurses who protested the changes were increasingly isolated from the new breed in their own ranks. Impatience with the individualism of public health's old spirit crept into the journal. In a debate over the proper nursing qualifications for venereal disease work, one nurse rejected her colleagues' elitism.

> It is well for us to remember that the work of the world is done by average persons. Many average nurses . . . can do more work and produce better results than a few very superior nurses. . . . We need to keep in mind that "top-notchers" have no corner on sympathetic understanding, on sincere interest in the welfare of others, or on obtaining cooperation.

Another writer criticized the independence of public-health nursing agencies as an obstacle to central planning.

> Intense, long-continued interest in a single nursing agency program is not easily shifted to equal devotion to community planning. It usually involves change in the attitude and sometimes the personnel of both the lay committee or board and the nurse administrator group.

Similarly, another nurse called for "a distinct change of attitude. . . . Here in the eastern seaboard particularly, voluntary agencies have been in danger of thinking of themselves as leaders because they were often pioneers." In sharp criticism of a new manual, *Public Health Nursing* itself attacked the old identity. The review reproved the author for putting "too much emphasis on . . . public health nursing as an entity or specialty rather than on . . . community nursing and the qualifications essential to every professional nurse to enable her to function in this broader community program."[60]

The composition of public-health nursing belied the democratic leveling that this language suggested. If anything, the field had become more exclusive. Those who set the standards in public-health nursing had never embraced their less educated sisters in private-duty or institutional work. Census data documented a steady increase in their educational qualifications. By 1950, 60 percent had postgraduate courses in public health. Over 20 percent held college degrees, at a time when only 12 percent of student nurses had had even a year of college work. The credential for public-health nursing remained in the postgraduate curriculum, although some hospital schools included a community health rotation in their diploma programs. Leaders resisted pressure to train all nurses for public-health work at the undergraduate level. In a rhetorical question that revealed much about the self-image of public-health nurses, one asked, "Shall We Teach Them All to Fly?" She answered with a firm negative. Public-health nurses represented a declining proportion of all nurses: in 1950, 25,000 counted themselves in the field, a little over 8 percent of all active nurses.[61]

If public-health nurses had been able to overcome their fear of dilution enough to recruit more widely among nurses, they may have been able to develop a more effective strategy for maintaining their independence. Instead, most seemed content to rely on their credentials and expertise, claims that would prove empty against the established authority of physicians. Eagerly responding to the new medical and public recognition of public health, many nurses seemed ready to accept the changing organization of their work.

The spirit of rationalization worked a pronounced change in the public-health nursing method, as the old balance of personal and "scientific" elements tipped towards a preoccupation with social science. By the 1940s, the reform spirit and the individual approach of the 1920s had largely evaporated. Nurses regarded their patients with new suspicion and explicitly rejected the maternal role of the old reformers. Freudian psychology and social work rationality recast nursing methods. Warning against over-dependence, one nurse explained:

> It is quite a usual thing to hear patients say, "You are like a mother to me," and many of them show the hurt feelings at the fancied neglect of themselves by the nurse which a

child will show when his mother appears to be giving more attention to one of the other children.

Others advised nurses to avoid becoming a "mother symbol" by maintaining the distance of professional demeanor. "The nurse's attitude to the client must always be impersonal without being patronizing; objective, yet subjective enough to understand the client's needs. A stronger emotional relationship cannot be had . . . without the work suffering." By the postwar years, the jargon of the social sciences had largely replaced social conscience and personal attachments. The "nurse, teacher, counselor, and friend" viewed her patients over a new clinical distance. As one nurse explained enthusiastically, "Nurses are learning to be experts in scientific friendships which make interpersonal relationships count for most." The crusading fervor of the public-health movement was gone, replaced by the brisk efficiency of the social engineers.[62]

After World War II, the voluntary public-health agencies lost their last sources of funding, largely due to the changing nature of public health itself. The death rates from contagious diseases had fallen dramatically; as more people survived to older ages, patients with chronic diseases increasingly dominated the case loads of the PHNAs and visiting nurses' associations. Demands for morbidity care rose sharply. In part, this reflected changes in hospital care: with shorter periods of hospitalization and new emphasis on out-patient treatment, more patients required home care from the agencies. For example, in the 1920s, tuberculosis patients spent months or even years in sanatoriums. With the use of new anti-tuberculosis drugs, these patients were quickly treated and released to home care. The new demands for nursing care largely indicated the different character of chronic disease and the limits of medical intervention. Doctors could offer little to patients with advanced cancer, heart disease, kidney failure, or complications of diabetes. Yet these patients did need nurses to give injections, plan diet, assist with routine care, and

provide moral support and occasional relief to families taxed
by long-term home care.[63]

Despite the pressing need for these services, the Red
Cross discontinued its support to public-health services in
June 1950, after almost four decades of funding rural and
visiting nurses' services. And in 1951, the Metropolitan Life
Insurance Company announced its impending withdrawal
from public-health nursing. As the incidence of chronic disease rose steadily, these groups undoubtedly feared the drain
of rising costs. Insurance companies, which had funded public-health services in hopes of preventing expensive illnesses or
early deaths, had little to gain from funding the care of chronic
patients. Larger social and cultural expectations of medicine
also militated against a broader commitment to chronic patients. By 1950, public-health workers could point with pride
to improved infant mortality rates and a healthier population
of school children. In mainstream medicine, doctors valued
and promoted aggressive medical and surgical intervention in
acute illness. Practitioners in preventive and curative medicine
alike were ill-prepared to meet the needs of patients who
suffered from intractable chronic diseases. Often beyond the
reach of medical miracles, the chronically ill could hope only
for temporary improvements, partial victories in a struggle
that most would lose to premature disability and death.

The public-health movement's propaganda for preventive care now became an argument against funding the voluntary agencies. As the Red Cross and Metropolitan Life backed
away, they echoed the maxims of preventive care that public-
health nurses had recited in the 1920s, and rejected the pallia-
tive care of chronic patients. The irony was not lost on public-
health nurses themselves. One nurse observed that the
public-health nurse "is almost oppressed by the time-honored
axiom that 'an ounce of prevention is worth a pound of
cure.' "[65] Set forth to expand funding for public health, the
argument was now deployed to close the doors on the growing population of the chronically ill.

Few voluntary agencies could raise enough money to

replace the insurance funding. When their Metropolitan Life contracts ended in January 1953, the 741 visiting nurse services affiliated with the company suffered an average budget cut of 10 percent. Four hundred nurses hired directly by Metropolitan Life lost their jobs. Of the 69 communities where Metropolitan had funded the only visiting nurse service, only 11 formed new agencies to take up the work. Attempts to raise money from local sources often failed, and in other places funding was so limited that services had to be cut back sharply. One agency's desperate expedient dramatized the hard times that had overtaken the PHNAs. Unable to pay full salaries to its nurses, the agency rotated nurses to staff jobs in local hospitals to supplement their incomes. Others tried to persuade hospital prepayment plans to cover visiting nurses' services. From tentative experiments with medical insurance in the 1930s, Blue Cross and Blue Shield were emerging to claim their central roles in postwar hospital expansion. But despite public-health nurses' efforts, insurance rarely extended to home nursing services. *Nursing Outlook* reported in 1954, "Administrators of the Blue Cross and Blue Shield insurance programs tell us they get no requests to include home nursing services as a benefit, except from the nurses themselves." In the early 1950s, many voluntary agencies surrendered their independence to combine with the better-funded official agencies.[66]

In 1953, the NOPHN dissolved itself, officially marking the end of public-health nursing's separate identity. After five years of debate, the NOPHN finally had accepted a two-organization plan for nursing. It merged with the prestigious National League of Nursing Education and the newer Association of Collegiate Schools of Nursing. In this regrouping, public-health nurses tacitly identified themselves with the nursing elites represented by the NLNE and the ACSN and symbolically reaffirmed their own special commitment to teaching and education. The reorganization had been achieved after a long battle in which NOPHN leaders struggled to preserve a shred of their old identity. They had refused to

merge with the American Nurses' Association because the
ANA would not accept lay members in full standing, violat-
ing the public-health commitment to a joint lay and professional organization. They won lay membership, but they also
surrendered their old autonomy within nursing. The
NOPHN was not even represented on the committee to set
the by-laws for the combined organization, the new National
League for Nursing (NLN).[67]

Public-health nurses gained and defended an elite position
within nursing without making any objective claim to superior scientific knowledge. Their reputation within nursing
rested partly on their educational credentials: as a group, public-health nurses did have more years of training than their
colleagues working in private duty or hospitals. But their
actual practice drew on knowledge and skills that all nurses
shared.

Indeed, public-health nursing could be seen as the least-
skilled branch of nursing, as it was the most tenuously linked
to medical science and technology. Despite the enthusiasm of
early reformers, the scientific advances of the late nineteenth
century generated few clear imperatives for everyday living.
While the vaccination campaigns and epidemiological research of the public-health movement offered new methods
for preventing and controlling outbreaks of disease, precipi-
tant declines in contagious disease mortality actually occurred
before these discoveries, thus deflating the movement's
clearest claim for the efficacy of the new science of health.
Infant mortality declined in the first three decades of the
twentieth century, and here the clean milk campaigns and the
attention to prenatal and early child care played a part. But the
scientific bases for home hygiene, nutrition, and child care,
which were the core of public-health programs, are still
poorly understood and still unformulated in the scientific
literature. Aside from its scientific rhetoric, public-health
nursing's approach closely resembled the pragmatic, com-

mon-sense practice of traditional lay nursing. Although Florence Nightingale adamantly rejected the germ theory, she would have thoroughly approved the public-health nurse of the 1920s and 1930s, with her emphasis on a clean, quiet, and healthy environment.[68]

The special prerogatives public-health nurses exercised on the job sprang from the social organization of their work: their exclusion from mainstream medicine and their organizational base in semi-autonomous agencies. In the 1920s and 1930s, nurses enjoyed the privileges of their isolation. Thanks to the agencies, they operated outside the usual constraints of relationships with doctors and patients. This fostered an innovative spirit: nurses pressed against the limits of traditional nursing practice to assert an independent relationship with patients. In joining the fight for preventive care, nurses also won a measure of independence for themselves.

But as outsiders, nurses had little impact on the institutions that ultimately controlled medical services. In its forty-one years in existence, the NOPHN helped to relocate public health from the outposts of rural counties and settlement houses to the hospitals, the growing centers of medical care. Once challenged by both physicians and laypersons, public health now settled into a respectable maturity. As public health gained acceptance, the medical profession asserted its control, barely ruffled by public-health nurses' former independence. At the same time, hospitals stripped public-health nursing of its innovative character, replacing home visiting and individual approach with rationalized care. As the institutions and practitioners of mainstream medicine embraced the public-health message, the nurse's special role was undercut. Newly converted to the gospel of health, doctors and hospital administrators overlooked its elite ministers to proclaim, in the words of a popular postwar slogan, "Every nurse a public health nurse."[69] The success of public-health nurses was an ironic one: they entered the elite center of medicine only at the cost of their autonomy.

CHAPTER 5

On the Ward: Hospital Nurses since 1930

In the 1930s, graduate nurses began to move from free-lance private duty to hospital staff jobs. Nursing practice took its modern form as hospitals hired increasing numbers of graduates for general ward duty. Once run by students or attendants supervised by a single graduate nurse, hospital wards rapidly became the province of graduates. The transition took place within the space of fifteen years. In 1927, nearly three-quarters of hospitals with training schools relied exclusively on students for ward nursing services; a decade later, most reported that they had begun to employ some graduate staff nurses. By 1940, nearly half of all nurses were employed in hospitals, and by the end of World War II, a decisive majority of active nurses held hospital jobs.[1]

Hospital employment had complex implications for nursing practice, creating a set of new possibilities and limits that reshaped nurses' experiences on the job. Exchanging freelance work for institutional employment, nurses discovered the decidedly mixed blessings of a bureaucratic work-place. They soon confronted the disadvantages of their new positions. Managerial innovations redesigned the hospital, changing its physical arrangement, the flow of work, the division of labor, even the performance of individual proce-dures. Nurses occupied an influential niche in the new order, but they also faced fundamental changes in their work, im-posed from above, which undermined traditional skills and ultimately threatened the very identity of nursing itself. Hos-pital nurses found themselves in the service of a Faustian bargain, for even as the work enhanced their opportunities

within the bureaucratic structure, it undercut both leaders'
hopes for professional autonomy and ordinary nurses' aspirations for craft control.

Yet despite the all-too-obvious problems of hospital
work, this new setting represented a distinct improvement for
nurses. Institutional jobs eased nurses' living and working
conditions, replacing the irregular work of private duty with a
modicum of security. The technological environment of the
hospital buttressed nurses' claims to special expertise. The
content and organization of hospital work gave nurses new
leverage in their relationships with patients and doctors. In the
ward setting, nurses gained the sociability and support of
small work groups; if hospitals imposed new constraints on
nurses, they also provided abundant resources for resisting
them. Most of all, nurses' expanding responsibilities and technical expertise supported a growing sense of entitlement that
led to new challenges to hospital management and medical
authority.

I. THE HOSPITAL IN TRANSITION

The move to graduate staffing was one phase in a larger
transformation in hospital management and in the organization of medical care. In the 1920s and 1930s, administrators
self-consciously introduced rationalization to the hospital,
drawing parallels between hospital care and industrial production. However, conflict among managers and resistance from
doctors and nurses indicated the persistence of older conceptions of hospital management, and even the most enthusiastic
rationalizers were careful to note that the principles of industrial management could not be transferred uncritically to the
hospital. As in other industries, scientific management was
used selectively and reinterpreted to fit the special circumstances of hospital work. But by the 1920s, efficiency and
rationalization were prominent management considerations
that were discussed often in hospital journals, and the chang-

ing face of the hospital reflected the assumptions and ideology of scientific management.

The rhetoric of efficiency was not altogether new. The "once-charitable institution," as David Rosner has called it, had already modified its philanthropic ethos with a business sensibility. As Rosner and others have suggested, considerations of order and discipline had begun to reshape American hospitals by the late nineteenth century. The concept of stewardship gradually gave way to more concrete principles of financial management as administrators sought a broader clientele and looked to patients' fees to underwrite a larger part of operating costs. Yet the decentralized character of hospitals made it difficult to apply industry-wide principles of rationalization, and managers themselves still held to an older conception of the hospital as a home, with a concomitant reliance on the paternalistic authority of the nineteenth-century family.[2]

By World War I, the scope of hospital care had expanded, and, with improvements in diagnosis and treatment that depended on sophisticated technology, hospitals extended their dominance over medical care. Doctors used hospitals more for private patients: surgery and childbirth, for example, took place at home less often, and even routine diagnostic procedures moved from home to hospital as equipment costs rose. By the 1930s, it was clear that private contributions and patients' fees could no longer cover the expenses of hospitals. At the same time, the local orientation of hospitals broadened. The wartime shortages of medical and nursing care, the influenza pandemic, and the initiatives of the public-health movement all created a national consciousness of medical resources and a new pressure for coordinated planning.

Managers gave new attention to the economies of scale that might be achieved through industry-wide planning. Industrial engineers began to appear on convention programs and in the journal of the American Hospital Association (AHA). At the 1926 AHA conference, for example, administrators heard a speaker from the U.S. Department of Commerce who described the principles of simplification and standardization and advised on their application in hospitals. He commended administrators' successful cooperation in standardizing hospital beds and china, and noted their progress in working for a common standard for sizing hospital linens. In the discussion, participants urged their colleagues to extend standardization of equipment to items like storage cabinets and door hardware. One committed simplifier reprimanded the renegades who ordered odd sizes and thus raised costs to the whole industry. Such reports revealed administrators' growing consciousness of hospitals as units in a national industry, not simply isolated philanthropic institutions or service institutions for local doctors and patients.[3]

Within hospitals, administrators rearranged the physical space to reflect new ideals of function. Once organized by class and gender, patients were increasingly sorted by their medical needs. The use of space in late nineteenth-century hospitals had reflected administrators' efforts to attract a paying clientele. The traditional common wards were bordered by private rooms; charity floors were flanked by private pavilions.[4] Under new imperatives of efficiency, space was allocated according to medical and nursing routines. Although hospitals did not become classless—private rooms and suites persisted—the overall design of hospitals emphasized their therapeutic purposes, with medical and surgical floors, obstetrical and gynecological wings, orthopedic units, and the like. Managers introduced more centralized services, reducing the functional autonomy of each floor or unit to streamline the flow of materials throughout the hospital. Central kitchens concocted the special diets that had once been prepared on each ward. Central supply services took over the floor nurses' old tasks of preparing dressings and sterilizing equipment. Considerations of efficiency influenced floor plans, as analyses of ward traffic patterns suggested ways to save steps. Rationalization reached down to the most minute details of ward routine, as time-and-motion experts scrutinized everything from complex postoperative care to taking temperatures.[5]

The spirit of professionalization also overtook hospital managers. Like other aspiring professionals, they sought to create and enforce uniform standards for hospitals and worked to define their own work. In the late 1920s the AHA instituted a system of voluntary accrediting administered by the American College of Surgeons. Administrators began to define hospital management as a distinct specialty, working to impose some uniformity on a diffuse and ill-defined occupational category. Doctors and nurses dominated the field, suggesting the conception of hospital management as an extension of medical and nursing routines. But laypersons had begun to take command of the larger and more diversified operations, indicating a developing consciousness of hospitals as businesses. In 1925, over 38 percent of general hospitals were headed by laypersons; doctors ran another 32 percent and nurses administered in 28 percent. Smaller hospitals were more likely to be run by doctors and nurses.[6]

Early proposals for administrative training envisioned hospital management as work that required both medical and business acumen. At a 1919 convention of the AHA, one member introduced a plan for a course of instruction in hospital management. The prospectus was directed to doctors, and the author, a physician himself, underlined the importance of familiarity with medical regimens. He also acknowledged the role that nurses had played as hospital managers and indicated that they too would be candidates for the administrative credential. In this conception, medical or nursing knowledge was no longer enough for good management—but it was still necessary.[7]

But the new administrative specialty quickly moved its emphasis from therapeutics to business management. The Rockefeller Foundation, a powerful sponsor of nursing and medical reorganization, was quick to underwrite these stirrings toward professionalization in hospital administration. In 1922 the foundation funded the Committee on the Training of Hospital Executives. Predictably, the push for a "professional" hospital administrator came to center on creating a restrictive credential. The committee recommended college-based education, a twelve- to eighteen-month course covering the equivalent of premedical requirements along with business electives, and a practical rotation. Subsequent programs began to resemble a business-oriented training. Proposed curriculums included courses in medicine, industrial engineering, and general business management; the program designers no longer assumed that candidates would be familiar with medical or nursing regimens. While in fact the most likely candidates for such instruction were already working in hospital management positions, the program's sponsors looked toward the redefinition of hospital administration as a distinct specialty, with recruitment channeled through academic institutions. In 1933, the American College of Hospital Administrators formed to support the cause of university-based training, and the first college program opened in 1934.[8]

At first such proposals had little practical effect. In 1925, a follow-up article on the first three courses for administrators indicated that only one had been given; no one had signed up for two of the available programs. The author noted, "There is a universal recognition of the *need* for a trained hospital personnel, including the superintendent. There is doubt expressed as to the *demand* for trained administrators." Nonetheless, these early efforts to define a course of training indicated the influence of both professionalization and rationalization on hospital managers. As one AHA member declared,

> this is an age of specialties. We can follow it all along the line of business, in manufacturing, in labor and especially in the building trades, in farming and in the various professions. Any business today that is not headed by a trained man who can control lavish expenses, check false economies, inefficient purchasing, inadequate inspection, excessive labor turnover and general lack of system and method which is so essential to a successful business, is doomed to failure.

Long dominated by ideals of stewardship, hospital management was entering into a realm of special expertise constructed by the "science" of efficiency.[9]

This growing interest in rationalization led administrators to reassess the traditional organization of hospital staffs. While some were content with students or attendants, others began to perceive disadvantages in the system. A workforce comprised of student-apprentices and freelance special nurses did not facilitate the flexible personnel management that rationalizers strove to produce in other industries. Hospital nursing schools permitted optimal discipline, offering literally a captive source of nursing service. But such paternalism had its perils: managers had to supply in return room, board, laundry, and administrative services. They also faced growing pressure from nursing leaders to offer more academic opportunities and to reduce the amount of required ward work. Although students could be summarily dismissed for poor work or insubordination, the workforce could not be increased or decreased at will to accommodate fluctuating needs. Meanwhile, hospital managers had to rely on notoriously independent special nurses to supply the extra amenities that private patients demanded, or to cover acute care that was beyond the abilities of partly trained students.

Nursing leaders' arguments against the apprenticeship system gained a new hearing from administrators in the late 1920s and early 1930s. A whole series of cost studies reexamined the economy of the hospital schools, and although most found that student nursing services provided a slight economic advantage over graduate staffs, all recommended the transition to graduate nursing. Often sponsored by nursing leaders, the conclusions naturally reflected their long battle against apprenticeship. But the cost studies also used a broader definition of efficiency consistent with hospital managers' interest in rationalization and their own professional aspirations. Proponents of student staffs emphasized economy, discipline, and control; in this traditional conception, good nursing service was the product of a system of personal authority and close supervision. Supporters of graduate staffs stressed the superior quality of service provided by the fully trained worker, an argument that associated nursing with the special skills and internal discipline ascribed to professionals. In this view of administration, good nursing service was the product of good nurses. Seeking their own place in "an age of specialties," administrators became uneasy about the wisdom of a staff of apprentice nurses or untrained attendants. Moreover, concerned with system and method, managers might well have begun to question the amount of time and money invested in on-the-job training and the rate of turnover built into the system of student nursing services.[10]

At bottom, a nursing workforce of dispersed freelancers and student apprentices was increasingly inadequate to the demands of the industry. Private-duty nurses' harsh experience during the 1920s had already pointed to the underlying weakness of this organization. The depression brought the lesson home to hospital managers as the demand for hospital care and staff nursing services increased sharply during the economic crisis. Many middle-class patients could no longer afford the services of a special nurse at home or in the hospital, nor could they pay for hospital services. Small private hospitals closed down as their supply of paying patients dwindled, while voluntary hospitals staggered under heavy demands for their charity services. To compound the pressure, student enrollments fell off, as fewer families could afford to give up daughters' earnings for two or three years of training school. Most schools no longer paid stipends, and many had begun to charge tuition. Leaders' modest gains had made nursing school somewhat less accessible, so that when hard times came, it became a luxury that many could not afford.[11]

Meantime, the demand for nursing service increased inexorably. Hospitals moved to a more solid economic base as insurance and federal funding increased, and the hospital industry entered a new period of consolidation and expansion. The total number of hospitals dropped as smaller institutions failed. Existing plants grew bigger, and overall the number of hospital beds increased by the thousands. At the same time, nursing care became more intensive with new hospital designs. Blue Cross insurance covered stays in two-, three-, and four-bed rooms; many patients who could not have paid for expensive single rooms could now elect semiprivate accommodations. The funding reinforced the changing use of space in hospitals, hastening the redesign of the old twenty-five-, and thirty-bed wards. On the old wards, nurses had supervised twenty or more patients from a commanding position in a large room. As the wards broke into smaller units, usually off central halls, nurses had to scurry from room to room to keep patients in view.[12]

Responding to this reorganization and expansion, more administrators called on graduate nurses to staff hospital wards. For some hospitals, the depression had shifted the economic advantage toward graduate staffing. Nursing leaders' constant agitation to decrease students' hours on duty had already constrained administrators' ability to collect in-kind service in exchange for training and maintenance. As hospital nurses' salaries were cut, some managers found that graduate services had become cheaper than maintaining their training schools. The cost studies done before the depression had shown that smaller hospitals in particular had operated schools on very narrow margins of profit. When patients fled from these institutions during the depression, some closed their schools, replacing their students with a smaller number of graduates. Elsewhere, shrinking student enrollments compelled administrators to look instead to the large pool of unemployed graduates. Managers benefited from the desperate straits of graduate nurses by instituting "work-sharing" plans, which enabled hospitals to increase their workforces without spending more. In these plans, hospitals converted to eight-hour shifts and divided two twelve-hour salaries among three nurses.[13]

However individual hospitals engineered the transition, the trend was far-reaching. In 1927, nearly three-quarters of the hospitals with training schools had relied exclusively on student services for ward duty. By 1937, 90 percent of these institutions hired graduate nurses to supplement their student staffs. Between 1929 and 1937, the ranks of general-duty nurses had swelled from 4,000 to 27,000. Nurses had always been closely tied to hospitals, products of the special experience and environment of the diploma schools. From the late 1930s on, most would never leave them: after they served their apprenticeships in hospital schools, they would spend their working lives as hospital employees.[14]

II. THE STOPWATCH, THE EFFICIENCY EXPERT,
AND THE NURSE

The emerging style of management revised nurses' experiences and prospects as workers, forcing adjustments in both professional ideology and craft traditions. Rationalization posed certain threats to both aspiring professionals and nurses on the job. Bureaucratic organization divided authority and responsibility in ways that compromised leaders' hopes of professional autonomy. In hospital jobs, nurses would be subject to lay administrators, the new experts, even as they continued to wrestle with the traditional restraints of medical authority. On the job, superintendents saw their old control erode as they lost their malleable student or attendant staffs. Graduates benefited from the decline of paternalistic discipline; at the same time, though, they faced intrusions on their own control, as managers imposed a functional division of labor that eclipsed traditional craft methods. But as they responded to the changes wrought by rationalization, nursing leaders and others again found themselves deeply divided.

By and large, leaders allied themselves with those hospital managers who turned to rationalization. They understood the expanding role of hospitals in medical care, and saw them as a strategic location for nurses. From their perspective, hospital nursing promised to remove two longstanding obstacles to professionalization. First, graduate staffing would release students from the apprenticeship system of the training schools; second, hospital employment promised a more secure and prestigious place for nurses, an alternative to the faltering private-duty market. Although rationalization did compromise the ideal of unconstrained professional autonomy, most leaders responded pragmatically, using the techniques and rhetoric of scientific management to strengthen nurses' authority in hospitals. Leaders sought to locate nurses at the fulcrum of the hospital's internal administration. They worked actively to delegate bedside nursing to other workers and to claim supervisory positions for nurses.[15]

Traditional superintendents and ordinary nurses, on the other hand, were considerably less sanguine about the emerging order. In the 1928 Burgess report, the overwhelming majority of superintendents declared their preference for student staffs.[16] New managerial strategies reduced superintendents' autocratic control over ward work, even as graduate staffs defied paternalistic discipline. On their own parts, many graduates also balked at taking their places in the proposed reorganization. Loath to give up the hope of independence that private duty represented even in its decline, they accepted hospital employment only reluctantly. Once on the wards, they resisted autocratic supervision and the sweeping control of the "total institution" of their nursing-school days. As institutional demands changed the content of their work, they protested the work pace and division of labor imposed by efficiency-minded managers.

Set against graduate staffing, superintendents illustrated the distance between traditional nursing services and the emerging bureaucracies of rationalized management. Supervisors were accustomed to exercising unquestioned authority, whether in the training schools or in hospitals without schools (where they managed subsidiary workers). The introduction of a graduate staff threatened to diffuse this concentrated authority. Neither apprentices nor "nonprofessionals," graduates were fully trained nurses who might disrupt the clear hierarchy of the accepted order. Superintendents feared that graduates would reject their strict discipline and worried that such insubordination would dilute their own absolute authority over students. In their eyes, special nurses had raised the same threat, and superintendents had moved to control subversive influences by isolating private-duty nurses in separate sitting rooms and dining rooms. But managing permanent, salaried nurses assigned to ward duty posed a more formidable challenge.

As hospitals began to hire graduates, nursing superintendents defended their traditional prerogatives as they complained about intransigent graduates. One rebuked graduates in her praise of the more compliant student staff: "Perhaps it is easier to manage; certainly it is more amenable to correction and discipline." The same nurse bemoaned the graduate's influence on impressionable students. "The student has set before her an example which we do not wish her to copy, but which she invariably does." Complaints about graduates' carelessness were so common that one suspects that they may have reflected supervisors' annoyance at variations in method rather than actual errors. "I don't know what gets into the nurses when they graduate," confessed one exasperated superintendent. "They seem to think that their diplomas are a license to discard every routine and technique they ever learned." Graduates also plagued their superiors by quitting regularly. "They have no sense of loyalty," wrote one superintendent with disapproval, and another corroborated, "They come with an 'I'll stay if I like it' attitude and leave as soon as something happens that doesn't suit them."[17]

Before 1930, hospital superintendents had enjoyed a degree of control that recalled the broad authority of the foreman in the traditional factory. Like the old foremen, they managed workers with little or no direct supervision from above. They hired attendants and admitted students, dismissed unsatisfactory workers, managed schedules of duty, imposed discipline, set standards of dress and demeanor. As Daniel Nelson has argued, scientific management in the factory chipped away at the foreman's prerogatives, limiting his personal authority and investing control in new departments removed from the shop floor. Hospitals, too, moved toward a more bureaucratic organization of management. New administrative schemes separated apprentices from workers and mediated the relationship of superintendent and staff through personnel departments and non-nurse managers. The developing system did imply a loss of power for superintendents: rationalization was transforming these traditional autocrats into middle-level bureaucrats.[18]

In the 1930s, staff nurses found themselves buffeted between traditional paternalism and the developing bureaucratic order. In many ways they experienced the worst of both worlds. Superintendents often continued to enforce the strict work and social discipline that they had applied to student nurses and attendant staffs. Hiring practices remained irregular; on-the-job supervision was frequently arbitrary and autocratic. At the same time, the rational discipline of scientific management began to make its mark in one hospital after another. The stopwatch and the efficiency expert symbolized the advent of a new style of management. Graduates found their traditional craft methods challenged by time-and-motion study data, and managers used notions of efficiency to press forward a more elaborate and rigid division of labor.

For graduates, hospital work seemed to spell the end of the craft control that private duty had symbolized. Nurses held out tenaciously against the rigid schedules and imposed discipline of institutional life. Registries reported that their nurses refused to take calls for floor nursing, and surveys indicated that recent graduates avoided hospital work. Nurses who were already employed on hospital staffs reported that they were seeking other work. High rates of turnover provided another measure of nurses' dissatisfaction.[19]

Before 1940, hospital employment probably offered little more security than private duty. Some evidence suggests that managers used graduates as a kind of reserve labor supply, exploiting the flexibility afforded by a large pool of unemployed nurses. Although superintendents might complain when graduates quit suddenly, they did not hesitate to dismiss their nurses on short notice. Unprotected by labor unions and vulnerable in the severe unemployment of the depression, graduates sometimes found themselves summarily fired. An examination of hiring practices at seventy-five hospitals documented the job insecurity that graduate staff nurses faced. Fifty-six of these institutions hired nurses with no specific guarantee of the job's duration. Of the nineteen that stated some definite term, varying from one month to a year, only five offered their employees written contracts. As one nurse reported bitterly, the hospitals "expect you to take care of six or eight patients and as soon as they can get along without you, you are dropped." Mandatory unpaid "vacations" or indefinite layoffs were common hospital expedients for economizing on nursing service in slack times. Some hospital registries exerted pressure on their private-duty nurses to fill in staffs. One graduate wrote to complain that her hospital dropped nurses from the registry unless they accepted such temporary floor duty on a per diem basis whenever the hospital needed extra help. An editorial note acknowledged other reports of such practices. Under circumstances like these, hospital employment probably held few inducements even for embattled private-duty nurses.[20]

The living and working conditions of staff nurses presented other serious disadvantages. Through the 1930s, hospital employment meant a return to the paternalistic regimen of the training schools. On the ward, superintendents tried to apply the same strict discipline to both graduates and students. Most hospital administrators expected their nurses to live in the nursing residences. A 1936 survey showed that 84 percent of hospitals included room, board, and laundry as part of the nurse's wages. Even where institutional policy did not require nurses to live in hospital quarters, few administrators adjusted the salaries of those who wished to "live out." The uniformly low wages compelled many to use institutional residences. Nurses frequently complained about this arrangement, rejecting the confinement of hospital quarters and the curfews and social restrictions that had ruled their student days. As one letter noted, "The young women of today are accustomed to 'enjoy the privileges' of independent living. . . . Nurses . . . chafe under the inevitable restraints and irritations of constant supervision." Graduates defended their dignity at work and demanded more privacy in their personal lives. Even student nurses had begun to rebel against the ritual humiliation that was part of their apprenticeship; as graduates, young women vigorously resisted hospital policies that regulated their social lives and constrained their work.[21]

New techniques of scientific management introduced other threats to staff nurses' autonomy. Based on Frederick Winslow Taylor's methods, the movement for "efficiency" aimed to simplify production by reducing each task to its smallest components. Analyzing the minute components of the work, "efficiency experts" pared away at "wasted" motions and substituted the simplest methods. The resulting standardization of work disrupted the traditional craft process in many industries, often stripping workers of their skills and their control over production. Taylorization also lent the materials and the rationale for an increasingly elaborate division of labor. Once analyzed into separate components, the work process could be divided among a number of workers, each assigned to a few repetitive tasks. In nursing, as in other work, the actual application of scientific management was partial and incomplete. Most efforts to standardize nursing procedures, for example, ended in dismal failure. Nonetheless, the rhetoric of efficiency brought critical changes to the pace and organization of hospital work. As defined by rationalizers, "efficiency" placed a premium on speed, which encroached on traditional craft practices in nursing. Although the analyses of efficiency experts never produced a reliable measure of nursing skill, managers still invoked the principles of rationalization to justify the extended use of auxiliaries.

Both professional leaders and nurses on the job struggled to control and direct the reorganization of hospital nursing. Although leaders sometimes disagreed among themselves

over the proper uses of scientific management, they accepted
the underlying logic of efficiency and ultimately supported the
increasing division of labor that accompanied rationalization.
Nurses on the job were more wary of the new techniques, and
many criticized leaders' gradual acquiescence. Staff nurses did
benefit from some of the changes instituted by efficiency
experts, and sometimes they themselves initiated studies to
evaluate and revise their own work. But more often, these
nurses experienced rationalization as an imposition. Protesting the new authority of the stopwatch, nurses tried to claim
control over the pace and content of their work.

Reflecting leaders' attitudes toward scientific management, the *American Journal of Nursing* generally emphasized
the benefits that nurses might derive from rationalization. The
journal reported enthusiastically on the use of scientific management to shape a more convenient and safer workplace. One
study, for example, analyzed accidents on hospital wards,
offered recommendations for safer nursing techniques, and
urged administrators to correct hazardous conditions. Other
articles praised rationalized arrangements that lightened the
physical effort of nursing. "Study Your Troubles!" exhorted
one author, in an article that explained how to save steps for
nurses on the wards. Similarly, the journal noted the conven-
ience of central supply services and diet kitchens.[22]

In its coverage of efficiency studies, *AJN* conveyed leaders' hopes of using the tools of scientific management to
improve nurses' working conditions and to enhance their
authority. The journal described two early time studies done
in obstetrical and pediatric units at two hospitals; nurses in
those institutions used their data to demonstrate the need for
more staff nurses. The NLNE itself used time study to argue
for better staffing and shorter hours. In a 1936 survey, they
timed a range of nursing procedures; calling on the authority
of this data, they calculated appropriate nurse-patient ratios
and condemned understaffing as "inefficient."[23]

Articles in *AJN* also promoted streamlining and standardization of procedures. The journal provided approving

reports of such efficiency measures, accompanied by detailed directions for replicating the studies. Initially such analyses were used to break down the resistance to graduate staffs, for it was only with the introduction of "outside" nurses that variation in technique had become an issue. In hospitals where students carried the nursing service, the school's time-honored methods were practiced religiously throughout the wards. But as hospitals began to hire more graduates, the automatic standardization of the old student staffs evaporated. Accustomed to her own school's protocols, an "outside" nurse might search in vain for supplies which her new workplace did not use, or fumble in assisting a doctor because a familiar procedure was performed differently. The journal documented a brief burst of enthusiasm for strict standardization of procedures. Proponents joined rationalizers in the quixotic quest for "the one best way," aiming to perform time studies on each of hundreds of procedures and then to set a single standard technique that all the training schools could teach. Such precise standardization proved wildly impractical. Nurses used hundreds of procedures that changed constantly with medical innovations and modifications in equipment. And patients provided an uncontrollable source of variation, confounding rationalizers with their nonstandard anatomies, idiosyncratic diseases, and unpredictable responses to treatment. Nonetheless, the doomed effort to organize uniformity in procedures demonstrated leaders' eagerness to mold nurses to the perceived requirements of hospital jobs.[24]

Nurses on the job viewed rationalization with a more skeptical eye. While journal reports emphasized the bright potential of scientific management, ward experience had schooled ordinary nurses in its actual applications. In theory, rationalized methods derived from time study could make work less fatiguing; in practice, managers applied it to require increased production from each worker. Hospital nurses lived out a reality that was seldom acknowledged in leaders' visions of scientific management. Administrators looked to rationalization for a simple and cheap solution to labor shortages, and

nurses learned quickly that "efficiency" was often synony-
mous with speed-up. "It takes young legs to keep up with the
pressure and speed. . . . Sometimes nurses do more 'things' in
one hour, new tests, treatments, etc., than we older women
used to do in six hours." Another complained that her friend
had to give evening care to fourteen patients in an hour, while
another colleague rushed through a patient's specialized postoperative care in six minutes. "Even the younger . . . general
duty nurse is breaking under the strain, and still the surveys go
on with the slogan 'Greater Efficiency!'" Other nurses explicitly criticized the use of scientific management to stretch out
increased work over smaller staffs. As one nurse insisted,
"The employment of more graduate nurses in our hospitals to
care for patients on general duty will do for us what we have
not permitted efficiency experts to do."[25]

Less tangible considerations of craft also informed ordinary nurses' resistance to rationalization. Nurses on the job
sometimes refused to follow revised procedures, defending
the venerable traditions they had learned in training school.
For these women, nursing methods were more than the
rational means to efficient performances: they also represented
their ties with their schools, and the training and experience
behind their hard-won skills. Transplanted from their alma
maters to alien hospitals, graduates asserted the traditional
localism of the schools by a fierce pride in their original
training. As one superintendent noted,

> The conflict of loyalties is something very real. One
> graduate nurse said "she felt like a traitor to her teacher"
> when she tried to use any other method than the one she
> had been trained to use. There are more arguments, more
> heated discussions, even more ill temper about trivial
> points of method than about almost anything else.

As graduates clung stubbornly to the protocols of their different training schools, superintendents despaired of enforcing
standard methods even within one hospital. The author

quoted above condemned the "provincialism" bred by strong alumnae associations. From a different perspective, her description provides a glimpse of nurses' craft consciousness on the job: they evoked the authority of apprenticeship traditions to defend their individual methods.[26]

Nurses called on a craft-based notion of good work to challenge the narrow definition of efficiency that guided scientific managers. *Trained Nurse* and *RN* both expressed a more measured and critical view of rationalization in their articles and editorials, countering the generally positive tone of *AJN*. Editorials warned that standardization of procedures might reduce nurses to being mere technicians, mechanical and unthinking. In letters to *AJN*, veterans of private duty protested that the art of bedside nursing was deteriorating as hospitals embraced industrial notions of efficiency. "We surely *lose* private duty *attitude*," one nurse wrote, "as we must rush everything through in a slam-bang way; checking off of duties assigned to us seems more important than the care of patients." Another letter portrayed the plight of former private-duty nurses who were exhausted and discontented in hospital jobs. "They are private-duty-minded, where everything you do for the patient's comfort is important, and have not learned to adjust to the general duty standards of essential care, consequently they do not get any satisfaction out of that type of nursing." By the 1940s and 1950s, most nurses would no longer have the experience of private duty as a reference point. Nonetheless, the basic issue of nursing craft would support an increasingly articulate protest against hospital work.[27]

The growing division of labor in hospitals was perhaps the most important outcome of managers' use of principles of rationalization. For years, both aspiring professionals and ordinary nurses had worried about the role of auxiliary workers, fearing that competitors without formal training would undercut the private-duty market and threaten the place of the graduate nurse. Nursing's leadership had vacillated between hoping to get rid of auxiliaries altogether and struggling to formulate licensing laws that would define and contain their

work. Meanwhile, hospitals had long depended on an informal division of labor, using non-nurse attendants or student
nurses to carry out the ward work under the supervision of
advanced students or graduates. Rationalization articulated a
theory that affirmed this division of labor; time-and-motion
studies and functional analyses provided methods for extending the division of labor and introducing formal new catego-
ries of workers. After 1940, leaders moved toward a more
decisive policy on auxiliaries, actively participating in the
development of practical nursing. With this shift, the different
orientations of leaders and nurses on the job were set into
sharp relief. Essentially, leaders accepted the redefinition of
nursing as a middle-management function, while ordinary
nurses remained wedded to older craft values, which placed
bedside nursing at the center of their work.

The "attendant question" had plagued leaders since the
inception of the professional associations. The persistence of
self-proclaimed nurses who lacked formal hospital training
was a galling reminder of nursing's incomplete professionalization. While doctors had gained the control over access to
practice that defines a profession, nursing leaders tried unsuc-
cessfully to create their own closed shop. In the 1920s and
1930s, some hoped to drive out these other workers, restricting all nursing-for-hire to those who held diplomas from
approved schools. The Burgess report warned that accepting a
"short course" nurse for private duty would only increase
"the servant girl element in the profession," and argued that
the attendants already working in hospitals should be replaced
by graduate nurses.[28] But the professional associations found
little support for this position outside of their own ranks.
Laypersons, physicians, and hospital managers favored the
use of auxiliary nursing services. In the 1930s, amidst declining student enrollments, overloaded hospital wards, and
strained finances, administrators increasingly turned to lower-
paid auxiliary workers to solve their staffing problems.

Signs appeared to indicate that leaders had begun to con-
cede to the pressure for auxiliary nurses, albeit with some

reluctance. In 1932, for example, the National League of Nursing Education agreed to develop guidelines for training aides and practical nurses if hospitals persisted in hiring them, although NLNE leaders reaffirmed their own commitment to all-graduate nursing staffs. Writers in the journals began to argue that nurses should accept the so-called practical nurses as a fact of life. Rather than trying to eliminate these workers, they suggested, the professional associations should assert control by incorporating subsidiary grades into a clearly defined nursing hierarchy. If nurses could not clear out auxiliaries, they could still defend their own positions by establishing and enforcing standards for the mandatory licensing of practical nurses. The NLNE's 1936 *Manual of the Essentials of Good Hospital Nursing*, by advising on the duties and supervision of auxiliaries, implicitly accepted subsidiary services. It advocated a flexible division of labor, based on skills or "functions" rather than on fixed tasks. For example, feeding a helpless patient might normally be considered a "non-nursing" task, properly the province of an attendant. But if the patient was "difficult"—upset, irascible, or very ill—the task might require the special skills and acumen of a graduate nurse. The NLNE strove to secure graduate nurses' control over the new division of labor: R.N.s would assign the work and thus set the limits of the auxiliary nurse's sphere.[29]

The journals left no room for doubt about the relative positions of the nurse and her subordinate. One nurse explained the division of labor in her hospital: "ward helpers" were restricted to certain well-defined duties, and clearly instructed about their lowly status in the nursing hierarchy. "She is made to feel that she is filling an important, though subsidiary, place in the hospital organization." Control of upward mobility also protected nurses against competition from auxiliaries. In the same hospital, good maids could be promoted to ward helpers, but these positions were considered permanent. As the author stressed, ward helpers were "regarded as *employees*, not *students*." Another nurse who described "the attendant's place" noted, "Several left to take up nursing, but we do not encourage it." This defensive posture persisted into the postwar years. A didactic short story written in 1948 portrays an exemplary practical nurse: she assures her supervising nurse, "I hadn't any notion of picking things up on the sly. Learning things I'd no right to be doing."[30]

If leaders remained cautious and defensive, ordinary nurses often felt even more immediately threatened by attendants. Some private-duty nurses blamed the inexorable decline of their work in the 1920s and 1930s on "irregulars." Although graduate nurses probably found more work in the shrinking market than their less-trained sisters, graduates felt understandably insecure about the ambiguous definition of nursing skills in private duty; they sometimes focused their resentment on practical nurses. On hospital staffs, working relationships among graduates and attendants underscored this ambiguity. As the NLNE had admitted, nursing skills were notoriously difficult to define with any precision. And whatever official definitions limited auxiliary work, on busy wards the staff exchanged and shared duties with a fluidity that further blurred the boundaries of the nurse's special expertise.[31]

Wartime mobilization increased the pressure on nursing officialdom to endorse auxiliaries. At first, professional associations parried public and federal demands for "nurse-power" with renewed efforts to rationalize hospital procedures, hoping to stretch existing staffs to meet the rising demands. These proposals delegated some "non-nursing" duties to practicals and aides, but the nursing associations still did not commit themselves to recruiting or training more subsidiary workers. As late as January 1941, both the ANA and the NLNE recommended that hospitals should hire only registered nurses for the direct patient care of bedside nursing.[32] With the outbreak of war, continuing shortages, and the possibility of a nurses' draft, the professional associations finally accepted auxiliaries as an official part of the nursing workforce. A three-point plan proposed in January 1943 included "the use of auxiliary nursing personnel for every function not requiring nursing skill," although even then the writer emphasized the use of temporary volunteers instead of paid workers. In December 1943, the National Nursing Council (the wartime coalition of the professional associations) formally capitulated to demands to mobilize paid auxiliaries. Public opinion and pressure had forced leaders to expand the nursing workforce; but even as they recruited practicals, they asserted professional prerogatives. A 1944 slogan expressed the reluctance of the nurses' concession: "A nurse for everything, but every nurse in her place!"[33]

Rank-and-file nurses received the decision with some misgivings. A report of the 1944 Biennial, the ANA's national conference, revealed that the delegates were far from unanimous in their support of the NNC's declaration. In a long discussion, some members questioned recruitment and training of practical nurses. An angry editorial in *Trained Nurse and Hospital Review* condemned the Council's unilateral action. "Overnight, the practical nurse was embraced. Nurses weren't asked—they were told. No other single event in my memory so shook nurses' faith."[34]

Nurses had always worked side by side with workers who had less formal training, but in the postwar years that division of labor became more clearly defined as auxiliary workers developed training courses and became more self-conscious and specialized. Uneasy about the emergence of formal training for practical nurses, some nurses on the job exhibited the narrow exclusivity that is part of both craft and professional culture. Just as doctors had feared competition from nurses in the early days of the hospital schools, so some nurses worked to set clear limits on the scope of the practical nurse's training and work. One nurse wrote the *American Journal of Nursing* to describe her district association's meeting, where members concurred that

a few months of training is enough for practical nurses. Such a program would prepare practical nurses to help professional nurses in caring for patients. But if women have a year or more of training they will not only take over bedside nursing, which rightfully belongs to the professional nurse, but they will sooner or later be placed in head nursing or even supervisory positions.

Others called for closer restriction of practical nurses' duties to protect the distinct status of the registered nurse. As one nurse demanded indignantly, "Why should students enter a three-year school of nursing, obtain an RN, and then find that practical nurses have the same privileges and rights?" Over and over again, nurses wrote to protest practical nurses' use of white uniforms and caps and even their claim on the label of "nurse." Instead, they suggested that licensed practical nurses (L.P.N.s) should wear uniforms that clearly distinguished them from three-year nurses, and that they should call themselves "trained attendants." Fearful of being displaced by cheaper workers with less training, nurses sometimes vented their insecurities in petty and divisive attacks on practicals.[35]

Leaders met their own fears of practical nurses' encroachment with a structural solution characteristic of professionalization. First, they moved to ratify and control the emerging division of labor. The ANA organized lobbying to pass state licensure for practical nurses, seeking a legal structure to assure and legitimate registered nurses' control over the nursing hierarchy. Leaders joined with hospital administrators and the young National Association for Practical Nurses' Education (NAPNE) to formulate accrediting standards. During the 1950s, licensing laws passed in state after state. Second, they sought a more restrictive credential for the registered nurse that would serve to curb mobility from below. The Brown report advocated a more rigid and permanent division of labor than had existed before: baccalaureate nurses would supervise and direct "technical" nurses and L.P.N.s.[36]

This proposed distinction between baccalaureate and technical nurses set off a storm of controversy. Many ordinary nurses declared war on their professional associations, or simply quit in disgust. Very likely the Brown report also exacerbated the tension between diploma nurses and L.P.N.s. As leaders implicitly devalued hospital-based training by portraying bedside nursing as menial manual labor, diploma nurses sometimes defended their skills by emphasizing their superiority to practical nurses. Also, the report represented the sealing of leaders' historical compromise with scientific management. They yielded to public opinion and to pressure from hospital administrators for cheaper workers in exchange for control of the developing nursing hierarchy. Faced with the problem of defining skill in an ambiguous context, they chose the professional solution—credentials. And recognizing that nursing's future lay in the hospital, they sought the leverage of middle-management positions.

Once again, as in their approach to nurses' education and to the private duty crisis, leaders showed an astute understanding of nurses' structural positions. To a great extent, their assessments of the possibilities of rationalization were borne out: nurses did gain skill and authority in hospital jobs. But in the volatile postwar years leaders also confronted unanticipated consequences of the division of work they had helped to define. As supervisors, nurses traded off many of the traditional compensations that bedside nursing had provided. Even as they advanced in the hospital hierarchy, their discontents multiplied. This time, they would reach outside the professional associations for help, forcing leaders to reexamine and redesign the agenda of professionalization.

III. HOSPITAL WORK AND THE REDEFINITION OF SKILL

The history of hospital nursing illustrates the complex implications of rationalization in service industries. On the one hand, nurses' situation seemed to replicate a familiar pattern: scientific management threatened to disrupt workers' control. Nurses responded like traditional craft workers, initially resisting the move to hospital work and cherishing the ideal of freelance independence. Certainly the impact of scientific management on the pace and organization of hospital work was far-reaching. Nurses felt a mounting sense of frustration with the pressure for speed and efficiency, and many expressed dissatisfaction with the fragmentation that came with functional division of labor.

But in other significant ways, the special character of nursing modified the meaning and consequences of rationalization. Nurses did not face the "degradation of work" described in Harry Braverman's stark *Labor and Monopoly Capital*.[37] Hospital jobs enhanced, rather than diluted, their skills. The expansion of medical knowledge added to nurses' technical virtuosity, and they gained status in patients' eyes by their association with the mysteries of advanced therapeutics. The social arrangements of hospital bureaucracy gave nurses the opportunity to negotiate more control in their relationships with doctors and patients. Finally, hospital nurses gained the support and camaraderie of a social workplace, an environment that fostered occupational solidarity and a sense of common interests and grievances.

After 1940, hospital nurses worked in a climate of expansion that contrasted dramatically with the decline and marginality of private duty. With Europe at war, Americans looked anxiously to medical and nursing resources at home; urgent calls for more nurses lent importance to the occupation and the women in it. During World War II, national recruiting campaigns and the debate over a nurses' draft further emphasized the critical role of nurses and nursing. Afterwards, the continuing expansion of hospitals outpaced the supply of nurses. The 1947 Hill-Burton Act provided generous funding for hospital construction, and postwar medical advances further increased the demand for skilled workers. As a result, nurses enjoyed a favorable labor market for the first time in decades. Hospital administrators desperately needed their skills and their labor, and, under the pressure of a national nursing shortage, they were forced to become more attentive to nurses' grievances about wages and working conditions.

Nurses' participation in World War II, especially in the

military at home and abroad, bolstered their authority in hospitals and in the eyes of the lay public. War propaganda stressed their competence and adaptability. Like campaigns designed to draw other women into war work, the appeals to nurses recruited them in the name of their traditional relationships to men, reminding the nurse that she was on the job as "the ambassador of all we left behind . . . our own mother, wife, sweetheart, or daughter." And even as nurses took on military rank with the responsibilities of command and endured the hardships of both domestic and foreign service, observers who commended their courage also insistently portrayed their femininity. As a sentimental male historian of nursing wrote in 1946, "Femininity in foxholes, with mud-caked khaki coveralls over pink panties, captured the imagination of the public and the fighting men of America." The campaigns were self-consciously aimed at mobilizing women only "for the duration," and thus the celebration of women's capabilities was tempered with reminders of the *real* woman's place at home. Nonetheless, the war's positive images of working women may have inadvertently helped women to gain a more enduring sense of competence and entitlement to work.[38]

The organization of war-time nursing also offered a dramatic model of a fully rationalized workforce. The graduate nurse took her place at the head of a more stratified nursing hierarchy. Commissioned as second lieutenants, military nurses had regular rank for the first time. In the services, they enjoyed the privileges of officers. On the ward, they supervised male medical corpsmen who did most of the bedside nursing. They outranked the corpsmen and the enlisted men who were their patients. At home, the widespread use of Red Cross volunteer aides and paid subsidiary workers forced nurses to define their own skills and to develop ways to use and supervise auxiliaries.[39] Physicians, laypersons, and nurses themselves adjusted to a new definition of the nurse's work and to the novel experience of female authority.

In the postwar years, new medical developments and

hospital reorganization enhanced nursing skills. As sophisticated technology supported greater intervention, and as graduate staffing led to improved nursing education, nurses gained practical skills and theoretical knowledge. Advances in critical care created a new division of nursing units that expanded nurses' skills. First was the "post-anesthesia" room, introduced in the late 1940s. Specialized postoperative care, once provided by special-duty nurses or staff nurses on wards, began to move to recovery rooms, where patients were treated until they revived from anesthesia. In the mid-1950s, hospitals began to organize medical and surgical intensive care units to segregate the sickest patients for concentrated care. By 1960, the term "progressive patient care" (PPC) indicated the spreading use of this organization. Patients migrated through intensive care, intermediate step-down units, and regular floors; or moved from surgery to recovery room to their wards. Further elaborations followed: the 1960s and 1970s saw the creation of dialysis centers, burn units, neonatal intensive care, specialized cancer wards. These changes produced nursing specialties, which were largely developed on the job. Nurses followed the proliferation of medical specialties and began to label themselves as intensive care, nephrology, or coronary care nurses. Nurses even prepared themselves to offer specialized care to those who slipped beyond the reach of therapeutics: the thanatology nurse worked to ease the last days for dying patients and their families.[40]

Progressive patient care illustrated the exceptional character of rationalization in medical care. Intensive care units were the response of hospital administrators to the new requirements of advanced therapeutics. Based on principles of rationalization, they were essentially a managerial innovation. Post-anesthesia units, first introduced in overseas military hospitals during World War II, were designed to concentrate specialized care in one area and to conserve skilled personnel. After the war, recovery rooms became an increasingly common feature in domestic hospitals. A 1949 description emphasized the efficient use of staff, with close attention to details of equipment and use of space. The author advised that patients should be arranged in two rows, with heads facing a central aisle. With this design, one nurse could supervise several patients closely and reach them quickly to intervene if necessary. Likewise, early reports of medical and surgical intensive care units (ICUs) stressed the advantages of concentrating highly skilled workers and expensive equipment in one area. Administrators saw ICUs as a solution to staffing problems, an innovation that would allow the best use of hospital nurses and that would lessen their reliance on private-duty nurses: some units even banned specials. Here managerial calculations went awry, for neither monitoring equipment nor spatial redesign effectively reduced staffing needs. Indeed, these units required larger numbers of workers: some even defined the ideal staffing as two to four nurses for each ICU bed. Moreover, moving the sickest patients to one area did not dilute the ordinary staff nurse's skill, for nursing care all over the hospital demanded new skills as medical intervention became more aggressive and treatments more complex. While staffing on the floor remained about the same, the specialized units caused the hospital's nursing workforce to expand.[41]

The hospital workplace and the changing character of medical care both improved nurses' positions vis-à-vis doctors and patients. Although nurses were often unhappy about the control that their institutional employers could wield, the bureaucratic and technological setting provided newly favorable conditions for managing medical colleagues and patients. Doctors experienced new constraints on their own work as their traditional entrepreneurial practice was modified by the changing institutional setting. Patients, too, had more limited control in the hospital as nurses escaped the personal service associated with private duty.

Hospital work significantly revised the conduct of nurses' relationships with doctors. Under these new conditions, the structure of medical authority remained the same: by law and custom, doctors were nurses' superiors. But in practice, doctors lost some of their economic and social control over nurses as private duty yielded to hospital work. In freelance work, nurses needed doctors' referrals to get and keep cases. A doctor who disliked a private-duty nurse's methods, manner, or even appearance could get her fired quickly. The nurse had no protection against such whims, and no recourse. Hospital nurses might still risk their jobs by repeatedly irritating or challenging a powerful doctor, but they were no longer directly dependent on the good will of any one physician.

The bureaucratic structure of the hospital diffused medical authority and offered nurses a modicum of support when conflicts arose with physicians. Doctors worked under the eyes of their peers and were subject, at least nominally, to the supervision and discipline of the medical chief of staff. The more public character of hospital work limited the physician's absolute authority. The private-duty nurse who questioned a doctor faced the consequences alone. In the hospital, a doubtful nurse could appeal to other knowledgeable participants, or invoke the impersonal authority of bureaucratic procedures and policies. Conflicts between nurses and doctors were still weighted in favor of physicians, but nurses gained a new leverage. Hospital nurses had the support of small work groups and the resource of a formal structure of appeal. Buttressed by her head nurse and sympathetic colleagues, a nurse could more readily confront a doctor on the floor. If informal approaches failed, she could take the conflict through established channels, and seek arbitration through the nursing director and the chief physician. Such procedures did not guarantee fair treatment, but they did provide nurses with a hearing. The postwar shortage of nurses and their important roles in the hospital also meant that administrators had a new stake in defending them. In one example, several surgical nurses resigned in protest against the hospital's irascible surgeons. The administrator persuaded them to stay and called in the medical chief of staff to discipline the doctors.[42]

Such incidents undoubtedly were exceptional, yet that they occurred at all testified to the benefits of nurses' new market positions.

Hospital nurses occupied strategic positions in the institution. The nurse commanded the domain of her ward: she knew how to negotiate the red tape of hospital rules, placate the patients, and get the work done. Learning to win the nurse's loyalty was part of an intern's initiation, and medical lore wryly acknowledged nurses' pivotal roles. A good nurse, every physician knew, could smooth his way as well as make his work more effective. Formally, of course, the nurse's duty was still to serve the doctor. But doctors who tried to enforce their prerogatives too insistently might find themselves stymied at every turn. Very secure nurses might risk the aggressive strategy of "forgetting" or simply ignoring a problematic order. In a safer (and probably more common) tactic, nurses could effectively hamstring a difficult doctor by working to rule: bringing him to the hospital at all hours by refusing verbal orders, invoking esoteric rules and procedures, inciting rebellion among his patients by refusing to discuss his plans or methods. Some obdurate doctors might persist in their folly, but most found it simpler to bend somewhat to the nurse's authority over the ward.[43]

Finally, the new content of medical care made nursing and medical work more interdependent. As advances in surgical and medical techniques promoted more aggressive medical intervention, the nurse's close observation became critical in the treatment of very sick patients. One nurse's narrative of patient care in the polio epidemic of the late 1940s offers a dramatic example. With careful observation, she detected a minute change in a young woman's breathing. Recognizing this as a sign of impending paralysis, she quickly called the attending doctor. The patient was placed in an iron lung, where she eventually recovered.[44] Nurses had always been responsible for close observation of their patients, and good nursing care had often determined the outcome in diseases like typhoid fever, scarlet fever, diphtheria, and pneumonia in the absence of effective medical treatment. But the development of new medical technology changed the significance of nursing observation and care in ways that brought nursing and medicine into a closer alliance. Twenty-five years before, when iron lungs were not yet in use, the nurse's observation would have signaled the limits of medical care; the physician could only watch helplessly and wait to sign the death certificate. Such a moment had a very different meaning and character as the possibilities for medical intervention expanded. Doctors depended on skilled nurses to watch for critical changes in their absence, and sometimes to initiate emergency treatment themselves. In this situation of close collaboration, doctors had to treat nurses more like medical colleagues.

Nowhere was this more apparent than in the mushrooming special care units, where nurses assumed many functions and responsibilities formerly reserved for physicians, and claimed a new authority by virtue of their expertise. The pace and character of intensive care left no room for the old formulas of nursing deference. No critical care nurse would call a doctor to report meekly, "Mr. Brown's pulse appears to have ceased." She would yell for emergency equipment, pound the patient's chest, inflate his lungs, initiate closed-chest cardiac massage, perhaps even begin to administer the drugs used in resuscitation. In turn, doctors recognized and depended on the skills and judgment of these nurses.[45]

Hospital employment also dramatically increased nurses' authority with patients. In managing the tasks and relationships of patient care, nurses had long recognized the advantages of the hospital as a workplace. Freelancers shunned hospital staff jobs, but they preferred to nurse their private cases in the hospital. Convenient facilities made the work easier, and a specialized workplace supported nurses' claims to skill and control over work. The private patient lost many old prerogatives, for in the hospital, nursing and medical considerations decisively outweighed lay preferences.

General-duty nurses slipped altogether beyond the reach

of the private-duty patient's dwindling authority, for they were employed by the hospital, not by the patient. Institutional nursing released nurses from the vestiges of personal service that clung to private duty. As one former private-duty nurse commented, "I don't have to entertain the patient and help trim last year's hat!"[46] Responsible for more than one patient, the nurse could limit the demands of any one person. She could excuse herself from one room to answer real or imaginary summons from another quarter, or seek a brief refuge from the entire floor by retreating to the nurses' station or the nurses' lounge. Working together, nurses also developed and enforced a shared prescription for the "good" patient. By disciplining patients to their proper roles, nurses avoided many of the disadvantages of private duty and could negotiate some respite from the quickening pace of hospital work. The well-schooled patient did not waste nurses' time with trivialities.

Fictional portrayals indicated the public's uneasy responses to the middle-class patient's new, humble status. Nurses might lack real autonomy at work, but they had gained enough authority to threaten cultural prescriptions for proper female behavior. In popular culture, the pathetic private-duty nurse of "Horsie" was replaced by more unsettling, if also more colorful, characters. "Hot Lips," the crack surgical nurse in $M\star A\star S\star H$, ran her nurses with an iron hand and kept doctors and enlisted men at a respectful distance. The formidable "Big Nurse" of Ken Kesey's *One Flew Over the Cuckoo's Nest*[47] policed her male patients to enforce her own version of order and discipline on the mental ward. In characterizations like these, the hospital world reordered the accustomed hierarchy of gender and class. Nurse characters gained a new and disquieting power, as their skills and authority at work reversed the proper dominance of men over women, upper-class over working-class people, customers over service workers. Dependent on the nurse, the sick patient had to surrender the usual prerogatives of social position.

Novels and short stories often showed male patients at

the mercy of their nurses. An especially striking example, a short story published in 1956, uses a patient's relationship with his nurse as a metaphor for the dependence and isolation of physical disability. T. K. Brown's prize-winning "A Drink of Water" explores the plight of a soldier who has lost his sight, his arms, and his legs in an explosion. While the fastidious critic or squeamish reader might rebel at this excess, the extreme situation of Fred MacCann effectively underscores his vulnerability. Fred must depend on his nurses to supply all his physical needs, to inform him about his surroundings, and indeed to mediate most of his action in the world. A gentle nurse gradually brings Fred out of his despair and grief. Although not too bright, she is good at anticipating his needs—to all appearances, in short, your ideal woman. Inevitably, Fred comes to adore the hands and voice that have saved him. The plot gains momentum as the nurse unexpectedly reciprocates and approaches him sexually. Delirious with surprise and gratitude, Fred finds himself in a torrid affair, and the two occupy their days in circumventing narrow-minded hospital authorities to drink and carry on in Fred's room. But one night the motherly-nurse-turned-seducer reveals another side of herself. To his horror, she breathes heavily into his ear and calls him her "man-thing." He realizes bitterly that the nurse's desire is not the affirmation of his intact humanity, but rather the ultimate objectification: to her he is only "a phallus on its small pedestal of flesh." He probes her past to confirm his dark suspicions. Just as he had feared, his beloved is a "man-hater": she can only love a helpless and mutilated man. Devastated, he kills himself, an act requiring no little ingenuity under the circumstances.[48]

In a world turned upside down, men lose their power to women, and women with unnatural power abuse it. This theme runs through postwar popular culture about nurses. Nurse-characters unbalance the proper relationships between men and women, alternately ordering men about and ignoring them; often asserting an unseemly sexual autonomy, either by seducing male patients or by abandoning them altogether for celibacy or lesbianism.[49]

Nonfictional sources echo this theme in more restrained criticisms of too-powerful nurses. A curious 1961 sociological study, "Authoritarianism in Nurses," purported to measure nurses' dictatorial leanings. Although the data failed to support the major hypothesis, the author concluded somewhat limply that, "nevertheless, the variable [authoritarianism] appears to be a significant attitude and personality dimension among the nurses sampled." In popular magazines laypersons denounced impersonal or "callous" nurses, and nurses themselves sometimes criticized officious or efficiency-minded colleagues. No doubt harried nurses on understaffed wards did sometimes become curt and impatient, and when they were forced to cut corners, they did not always have time to dispense "TLC" (tender loving care). But the tone of many comments about the new breed of nurses also suggests another interpretation: the nurse had grown too scientific and gained too much control of her patient to satisfy sentimental expectations of nursing as womanly duty.[50]

Bitter at the constraints of hospital jobs, nurses themselves might object to this portrayal of the advantages of an institutional workplace. Yet in historical context, hospital work did give nurses a stronger position in the labor market and on the job. They could and did exercise considerable control as individuals, picking and choosing their shifts and workplaces in a market desperate for their skills. On the ward, they claimed middle management positions, becoming the undisputed heads of the nursing hierarchy. In relationships with doctors and patients, they pressed the advantages of their new locations, challenging physicians' absolute authority and deflecting lay demands for personal service. These improvements did not constitute real control at work, and, in a wave of postwar protest, nurses outlined the many limitations of institutional jobs. But a historical perspective suggests that their dissatisfaction reflected more than the undeniable difficulties

of hospital work. Rather, hospital jobs supported rising expectations and facilitated collective action. Relocated from the
fringes to the center of medical care, nurses gained new responsibilities and began to demand a concomitant authority.

IV. STAFF NURSES IN REVOLT

Virtually as soon as hospitals began to employ nurses in
large numbers, general-duty nurses began to protest their
wages and working conditions and to articulate a sharp critique of hospital rationalization. Surveys and readers' letters
documented the disadvantages and discontents of staff nurses
in the late 1930s. The brand-new journal *RN* took up the cause
of "The Forgotten Woman" on general duty, urging the
ANA, hospital administrators, and laypersons to improve
hospital work. In the war and postwar years, the nursing
shortage gave staff nurses a new position of strength. In a
barrage of criticism, nurses prodded the ANA for more decisive action on their behalf, and an influential minority turned
toward labor unions. The issues dissatisfied nurses raised in
the 1940s and 1950s remain unresolved; today's coverage of
nurses in crisis recapitulates the themes of these earlier decades. But in the critical postwar years, nurses outlined a critique of hospital staff nursing that is still powerful today, and
began to move from informal resistance toward new forms of
collective action.[51]

With the postwar expansion, administrators scrambled to
find enough nurses to staff their wards. Physicians and laypersons raised the alarm about a "nursing shortage," a concern
that still dominates public discussion of nurses and nursing.
As the need for nurses increased, observers were newly concerned about the attrition rate in nursing schools and the large
numbers of inactive nurses. Analyses of the shortage often
emphasized the inevitable transience of nurses as workers: the
demands of marriage and motherhood, they argued, drew
nurses out of the workforce. In fact, a longer perspective
suggests just the opposite. Nurses, like other women, were

increasingly likely to remain on the job after marriage and to move in and out of the labor force as mothers. By 1951, 47 percent of all active nurses were married, compared to less than 20 percent in Burgess's 1928 report. But surveys of turnover sometimes did appear to confirm the notion that marriage and motherhood disrupted work: many nurses gave marriage, pregnancy, or home responsibilities as their reasons for quitting. The postwar ideology that was later named "the feminine mystique" urged women to go back to the home, and many feared that nurses were heeding the call.[52]

Nurses' angry responses to cries of "shortage" suggested a different interpretation. Intolerable working conditions and low wages explained the staffing crisis, they insisted. One male nurse wrote, "I strongly contend that there is no shortage of R.N.'s but only a shortage in their pay envelope. Get the salaries up where they belong and the whole trouble will disappear overnight." Others blamed the break-neck pace of ward work. "Institutions are short of nurses because they expect one nurse to do three nurses' work," a New York nurse explained bluntly, and a former general-duty nurse who had quit to become an industrial nurse corroborated, "The chief trouble with hospital nursing is that there is so much to do and so little time to do it well." The *American Journal of Nursing* acknowledged these widespread complaints in an editorial, advising "collaboration" among nurses, hospital administrators, doctors, and patients to improve hospital working conditions.[53]

Married nurses revealed another dimension of the shortage as they indignantly scored institutional rigidity. Hospitals complained of inactive nurses' refusal to pitch in at a time of national need, but they were not willing to modify their wage structure or hours to accommodate married women and mothers. Some hospitals continued to pay low wages supplemented by maintenance—room, board, and laundry— although such arrangements clearly discriminated against married women, and indeed against the growing numbers of single women who shunned institutional living. The trend did change rapidly. In 1936, 84 percent of hospitals included full maintenance in their salaries; by the end of 1946, less than 10 percent still required staff nurses to "live in," and most had made adjustments in salaries for "living out." Hospitals were slower to offer flexible working hours or part-time positions. One frustrated nurse told of her unsuccessful search for a general-duty job that would fit her schedule. "If hospitals are so desperately in need of RNs as they lead the world to believe," she remarked, "they could adjust the working hours so that a married nurse with children could work." Increasing numbers of women sought part-time work, but hospitals hired part-timers only reluctantly. Other nurses with children wrote to say they wanted to work but could not afford child care on hospital salaries. In the few hospitals that opened low-cost day nurseries, nurses returned to work with alacrity.[54]

Nurses also indicted hospital rationalization and division of labor. In a sustained editorial campaign, *RN* drew parallels between hospital and factory reorganization and portrayed the nursing shortage as an expression of nurses' dissatisfaction with rationalization. Postwar insurance fees and federal grants had funded capital expansion, not better salaries for more nurses; to meet the pressures, "Both patient and nurse went on the assembly line." Another editorial proclaimed, "The advances of science brought their own form of mass production, and mass production in health did to many nurses what mass production in industry did to many workers . . . destroyed the worker's sense of accomplishment. It came between the worker and the completed job."[55] Many nurses were unhappy with the growing division of labor and with their new administrative duties. As administrators increasingly placed registered nurses in supervisory positions, in charge of delegating bedside care to L.P.N.s and aides, many nurses regretted the loss of their traditional relationship with the patient. Before the days of "team" care, one recalled, "the satisfaction of seeing her efforts bring good results was hers alone." Paperwork and administrative tasks threatened to subsume traditional patient care; even in units with ward clerks, nurses spent more and more time directing the hospital's flow of paper, from approving requisitions for supplies to filing accident reports to filling out charts with endless notes of procedures and progress. One nurse wrote in despair, "Who can define a nurse? Once the answer was, 'One who is devoted to and tends the sick.' Today, an appropriate definition is almost impossible. To be accurate, you would have to say, 'one who keeps the records of the sick.' " In criticisms of scientific management, thoughtful nurses examined the quality of hospital work and many mourned "nursing's loss of identity."[56]

Finally, hospital nurses became more vocal in public criticism of medical and administrative hierarchies. Breaking the silence imposed by professional etiquette, nurses began to demand more recognition and respect from physicians. "The nursing profession could very well do without the shackles of autocracy enforced upon it by the MD and handed on down through the hospital staff." Infused with the passions of the recent war against fascism, buoyed by their own expanding skills and authority, nurses rejected the old militaristic order. "If democracy is good enough for other Americans to live by, it should be good enough for the medical profession." In other letters and surveys, many nurses agreed, and suggested that improved relationships between doctor and nurse might do much to alleviate the nursing shortage. Supervisors and administrators drew their own share of criticism. Janet Geister, a maverick nursing leader and longtime defender of private duty, wrote an impassioned editorial in *RN* castigating "Man's Inhumanity to Man," an indictment of the arbitrary discipline of hospital work. Her readers endorsed the sentiment emphatically. One noted bitterly, "Even a criminal has a right to a fair trial but not the nurse," and *RN* received a flood of letters and requests for reprints of the editorial. A few years later, in 1953, another aggrieved nurse demanded, "Why does an administrator speak of us as 'girls'? Why is it difficult or impossible for us to be heard when executives are discussing our problems and interests?" A staff nurse's letter poignantly conveyed the sense of impotence that many felt. "The basic difficulty is not money. . . . It is this feeling of being left out of all creative calculations and policy making which is discouraging."[57]

Unions were a controversial new approach to the problems of hospital nurses. In the 1930s, both the American Federation of Labor and the Congress of Industrial Organizations began to recruit among nurses, stirring considerable unease among professional leaders and the loyal opposition represented by the editors of *RN* and *Trained Nurse and Hospital Review*. In a 1937 statement, ANA leaders reiterated their longstanding policy against nurses' participation in labor unions, proclaiming the superiority of the professional associations. Nonetheless, a 1939 report estimated that probably five thousand nurses had rejected the ANA's advice in favor of a union card, and went on to describe the activities of strong nurses' unions in Seattle, San Francisco, and New York. The CIO had established locals in nine states in a campaign to extend the organizing drive among nurses.[58]

As unions recruited nurses into their ranks, some nurses reacted strongly against the notion of collective bargaining. Disapproving R.N.s reminded their union-minded colleagues of the guiding wisdom of the Nightingale pledge; collective bargaining, they argued, destroyed nursing's spirit of service and humanitarian dedication. "May God save us from that degradation!" one exclaimed. Nativist and class prejudice fed opposition to unions. A nurse from Seattle advised, "If one wants to be ruled by an alien who is practically illiterate, join a union and discover what real bondage means." After the war, a growing anti-labor sentiment probably reinforced the doubts of nurses like these. Despite widespread union cooperation during the war, many Americans, citing wartime strikes and agitation, felt that labor had not done its part. The 1947 Taft-Hartley Act placed new constraints on labor organizing. A series of investigations revealed corruption and undemocratic practices in some labor unions. The anti-Communist crusade of the 1950s poisoned the atmosphere, raising suspicions of subversion against even the mildest opposition politics. One nurse demanded, "Why should a nurse have to pay [union dues] to some gangster . . . ? This is still a free country, I hope," while another berated nurses' benighted interest in unions. "Will they forsake their civil liberties to become slaves to a dictator? Then, why give up their professional distinctions and become slaves to union leaders?"[59]

Yet other nurses expressed a growing interest in unions and collective bargaining—and a concomitant disillusionment with the professional associations. Like private-duty nurses who had challenged the traditional ideology of service, hospital nurses rejected pious exhortations about professional duty. As one nurse commented, "phrases such as 'professional prestige,' 'suffering humanity,' 'personal satisfaction,' and 'a grateful public' . . . do not compensate for any lack in the pay envelope. No butcher yet has accepted any one of them in payment for a pound of hamburger!" One letter exhorted, "I advise general duty nurses to leave the opiates of a super-professionalism and the sentimentality of an unrealistic florence nightingale-ism to their 'superiors' and get down to cases with their own interests. But don't count on the ANA." A Detroit nurse, rejecting the paternalism of hospital administrators, identified with a tradition of organized labor and with growing public-sector unionism. "The railroad men of our country have long had a 'brotherhood,' city employees, school teachers, and nurses in our county hospitals have learned that the big, happy family is happier with a bargaining agency." And others refused to see professional ideals and union activity as antithetical. Declared a New York nurse, "I'm proud to say I'm a good nurse and a good union member."[60]

Although only small numbers of nurses actually joined unions, the organizing drives directly influenced the ANA's response to general-duty nurses. The possibility of unionization gave discontented nurses a concrete alternative to the chronic surveys, self-analyses, and "upgradings" of the professional associations. Reports of successful negotiations set compelling results against the ANA's vague promises, and served to focus staff nurses' criticisms of the professional associations. The presence of labor organizers, and general duty nurses' often sympathetic responses, jolted the ANA into a stronger position of advocacy for staff nurses. Clearly it was no longer enough to assert the merits of professional associations: the ANA had to begin to deliver.

The response of the California State Nurses' Association (CSNA) presaged later ANA policy. The association began to work for improved wages and working conditions to keep nurses in the professional organization and out of unions. By 1942, California general-duty salaries were the highest in the country. The West Coast war boom was one explanation for this relative prosperity: hospital administrators had to raise wages to compete with lucrative jobs in defense industries. Very likely, they were also influenced by the growing interest in labor organization among nurses and the active AFL and CIO drives in hospitals. Administrators balked at direct negotiations with the CSNA; because the professional association was not a union, employers had no legal obligation to consider their demands. Frustrated members sought the legal structure of collective bargaining for the professional association. During the war, the CSNA moved into direct competition with the AFL and CIO drives, and in April 1943 the association won a representation election. The CSNA adopted a no-strike policy, as the AFL had also done, and continued to press their statewide platform to the Association of California Hospitals. Their "economic security program" stipulated minimum salaries without maintenance and laid out personnel policies on issues like scheduling, paid vacations, and health insurance benefits. Bringing the still-intransigent hospital administrators to the War Labor Board, California nurses finally won much of their program. In 1946, the ANA made the California example into national policy, announcing their own economic security program for nursing.[61]

After the tumultuous 1940s, collective bargaining had

relatively little direct impact on most nurses' work lives. Participation in the ANA's Economic Security Program was sparse and uneven. By 1960, only about 8,000 nurses were covered by a total of 75 contracts, and 74 of the agreements had been negotiated by just six state associations.[62] Internal conflicts and structural problems may have hampered the ANA's program. Many nurses remained mistrustful of the professional associations, and when the ANA raised dues in the 1950s to fund the Economic Security Program, membership dropped. Under the plan, state associations set policy and minimum standards for collective bargaining. This arrangement moderated the influence of a distant national organization, but also removed control from local district associations and from individual workplaces. The Economic Security Program labored under the inhibiting influence of its mixed constituency, for SNAs represented both supervisory and staff nurses. Superintendents had quashed private-duty rebellions in some district nursing associations in the 1920s and 1930s, and in the 1940s and 1950s they were hardly more willing to permit staff nurses to organize in their own ranks. General-duty nurses complained of intimidation when they raised the issue of collective bargaining.[63] Finally, until 1968 the ANA maintained its no-strike policy; state organizations had to depend on persuasion, a tactic that had never been notably effective with hospital administrators.

Labor unions also had limited success. The Economic Security Program probably deflected some nurses from unions; the ANA discouraged membership in both the association and a labor union, and the promise of support from a familiar organization may have kept some nurses in the ANA. The 1950s were moribund years for the labor movement in general, and neither service work nor women workers were traditional areas of union activity or strength. Strikes posed a special dilemma for nurses. If they relinquished the threat of withdrawing their labor, nurses negotiated from an untenable position. Yet hospital strikes raised serious ethical questions for many nurses, who agonized over refusing to care for the sick even as they defended their own rights as workers and fought for conditions that would improve patient care. Walkouts also created a tangle of tactical difficulties. Without a sustained public appeal, striking nurses were likely to find themselves isolated, as administrators won the support of an angry and uncomprehending community. Labor organizers themselves were not always receptive to nurses' concerns. Traditionally most effective with bread-and-butter issues, unionists sometimes gave short shrift to demands for better staffing or a stronger role in hospital decisionmaking. Perhaps most important of all, nurses' right to organize was not protected by law. The 1947 Taft-Hartley Act exempted voluntary hospitals from the National Labor Relations Act. Nurses' organizing efforts labored under that crippling handicap until 1974, when the exemption was finally revoked.

Labor organization fell far short of providing a solution to the many problems of hospital nursing, but it nonetheless improved some nurses' work and it altered the agenda of the ANA. Collective bargaining by unions or professional associations probably did have a ripple effect not visible in membership statistics or in the record of successful contracts. Especially in the context of an acute nursing shortage, hospitals clearly had a stake in keeping their wages competitive and their workers happy. Even more, the unions had changed nursing history by their appeals to the general-duty nurse. Staff nurses' dissatisfaction and the appearance of an alternative had pressed the ANA toward a more aggressive policy. Whatever its limitations, the Economic Security Program created a space within the professional association for activist nurses, and, in some places, nurses were able to negotiate collective bargaining agreements that raised wages and improved working conditions.

In the late 1950s and 1960s, the professional associations also began to respond belatedly to hospital nurses' critique of rationalization. The earlier emphasis on the nurse as manager became more muted. The journals still ran articles on standardization, simplification, supervision of auxiliaries, and unit organization, for management was now a staple of many nurses' work lives. But prescriptive literature also began to address issues raised by general-duty nurses and their advocates, struggling to recover nurses' distinctive identity and sense of mission within the context of a radically changed work setting. At least rhetorically, leaders showed signs of a reorientation to patient care.

Journals and textbooks emphasized the new concept of "total patient care," and portrayed the nurse as the hospital's bulwark against impersonality. Located in key positions, nurses could infuse bureaucratic regimens with the traditional concerns and intimacy of one-to-one nursing care. Total patient care embodied a telling contradiction, for, in this scheme, attending to the "whole patient" did not necessarily involve assigning each patient a whole nurse. Rather, the nurse was to take responsibility for coordinating care to avoid repetition and fragmentation. Total patient care, quickly abbreviated to TPC, was an effort to moderate the difficulties that arose with functional division of labor and at the same time to assert the nurse's special role on the health care "team." To some extent it was little more than a linguistic gloss that masked the thoroughgoing rationalization of nursing: as one graduate of the 1920s remarked, "We didn't talk about total care of the patient; we gave it." The new jargon of nursing theory sometimes recalled the empty phrases of public health's decline, when traditional patient relationships yielded to cold "scientific friendships." Rhetoric often flew blithely over real constraints. Without more substantive changes in the pace and organization of work, even the most dedicated nurses would have been hard pressed to approach the ideal that TPC expressed. Still, the renewed emphasis on patient care indicated a significant shift in leaders' approach to hospital work: TPC represented a tacit admission that the promises of rationalization had somehow gone sour. The new concern for the patient's experience also reflected consumer critiques. TPC was an attempt to revive an image of the hospital as a home for the sick, not simply a repair shop for the malfunctioning body.[64]

A welter of conceptual innovations in nursing theory followed, all aiming to redefine and strengthen the hospital nurse's relationship with her patient. In the 1950s, journals and nursing schools showed a renewed interest in the case method, which restored the craft organization of work to nursing care and teaching. Under the case method, one nurse would take responsibility for some number of patients, seeing to all their needs. Ideally, the same nurse would follow a patient from admission to discharge, coordinating care from shift to shift and giving the patient one element of continuity over the course of a hospital stay. In schools using the case method, students worked from the specifics of a single patient's illness toward the body of related knowledge, rather than beginning with abstract conditions and then seeking out representative patients. Case studies became a regular feature of nursing journals in the 1960s. Nurses would describe the care of a single patient in narratives that, while providing technical information about treatment, strongly emphasized the social and psychological dimensions of nursing care.[65]

Nurses also worked to find institutional forms for the renewed commitment to care that reflected older craft organization. "Primary nursing," for example, called for a new structure of assignments and record-keeping based on the case method. The primary nurse had the explicit responsibility of assessing and evaluating each of her patients' care. Others might give that care at times; primary nursing could accommodate some rotation of assignments. But it emphasized one nurse's ongoing relationship with a patient and affirmed the important role of direct contact and "hands-on" care, thus countering functional division of labor. Most recently, nurses have begun to struggle to create a career ladder for bedside nursing. The "nurse-clinician" can advance without leaving patient care behind, providing a new alternative in a structure that has long rewarded only supervisory roles and thus implicitly devalued bedside care. In elaborating the role of the nurse-clinician, nurses rejected the definition of bedside care as unskilled and redefined it as one among many nursing specialties.[66]

Yet by 1970, many nurses had become cynical about the possibilities of change, whether through the structure of collective bargaining or in the rhetoric of a revived commitment to patient care. The gap between young nurses' expectations and their experience became a recognized syndrome of occupational life. The new collegiate nursing schools touted the nurse's authority and encouraged her to be an active advocate for her patients. But once on the ward, she slammed up against the limits of hospital bureaucracy, medical authority, and inadequate supplies and staffing. After this rude awakening, which one observer called "reality shock," disillusioned nurses sometimes left nursing altogether or drastically lowered their expectations.[67] There would be no easy solution for nursing's dilemmas. But both professional ideology and apprenticeship culture contained possibilities that nurses have not yet fully explored.

Conclusion

The tension between nursing's two cultures still underlies and informs nurses' efforts to define and control their work. Leaders have gradually won much of their program; yet as more and more nurses earn degrees, they are discovering the limits of credentials as a means to gain the prerogatives of professionals. On the job, the culture of apprenticeship continued to reproduce itself and, in somewhat altered forms, the values of apprenticeship still flourish. The divisions introduced by the transition to baccalaureate requirements are not yet mended, and nurses confront the persistent limits of their work under the handicap of internal conflict and turmoil. But at the same, the traditions of professional ideology and apprenticeship culture each provide resources for moving forward nurses' claims to authority at work.

After the 1948 Brown report, the transition to collegiate education proceeded slowly but inexorably. New programs began to form and to recruit growing numbers of candidates. In 1952, the first associate degree program opened, offering an intermediate credential intended to rank between the hospital diploma and the baccalaureate degree. Associate degree nurses attended two years of junior college and took some clinical training. By 1963, these programs claimed a modest 4 percent of all new graduates. Baccalaureate programs increased slowly in number and influence, representing 14 percent of new nurses in 1962. In 1965, the professional associations took drastic action to speed the transition, setting a twenty-year deadline for the goal of a college education for every nurse. A small group of nurses passed the proposal without consulting the general membership, and inadequate provisions for diploma nurses provoked sharp antagonism and opposition. After the 1965 resolutions, nurses' education shifted decisively away from the hospital schools. More hospital schools closed each year, and by 1970 associate programs claimed over 26 percent of the new graduates, while another 20 percent held baccalaureate degrees. College-based programs were making headway in nurses' education and beginning to have an impact on their work lives: more and more supervisory or specialized nursing posts required the degree.[1]

Equally striking, though, was the persistence of apprenticeship culture in nurses' workplaces. Long after leaders proclaimed the superiority of the college-educated nurse, hospital school graduates often enforced another standard on the job. Schooled to appreciate firm control and practiced skills, diploma nurses scorned their uncertain and fumbling sisters, who came to their first jobs with degrees but also with less clinical experience. In the informal hierarchy among nurses, the degree nurse might have to humble herself to the hospital graduate. Baccalaureate nurses defended themselves in language that suggests their precarious status in workplaces still dominated by the values of apprenticeship. In 1969, for example, one college-educated nurse wrote *RN* to complain about the many letters that disparaged baccalaureate nurses. "A layman reading these letters would hesitate before allowing a BSN to trim his fingernails," she exclaimed. pleading for a fair hearing from diploma nurses: "I'm tired of being judged as unqualified simply because a few other BSNs haven't measured up. Let each of us be judged individually. I don't believe in condemning a whole group because of the faults of a few." As late as 1970, another college-educated nurse felt it necessary to remind intransigent supporters of hospital schools that "a degree nurse must pass the same state board exam as a diploma nurse. . . . our degree nurses need a *boost* instead of a *boot*."[2]

Hospital hiring practices sometimes enforced traditional standards of apprenticeship, for some nurse-employers treated the degree as a detriment rather than a credential. In one example, the American Nurses' Association demanded equal pay for associate degree nurses, who were being hired for lower wages than hospital school graduates in Minnesota hospitals in 1967. A 1976 state survey of 77 hospitals and 34 nursing homes in Kansas found that nurse-employers did not favor the nurse with a degree. Nurse-superintendents in hospitals of 100 or fewer beds frankly preferred the diploma nurse. In larger hospitals, nurses in charge of hiring considered the diploma nurse to be the equal of a baccalaureate nurse and superior to the nurse with an associate degree. The military concurred. The Army Nurse Corps refused associate degree nurses until 1971; the Air Force Nurse Corps did not relent until a year later.[3]

The vigor and resilience of ordinary nurses' work culture suggest a vision that might shape nursing's future. Apprenticeship culture has provided an alternative to professional ideology, a different structure within which nurses can affirm their skills and define their work. In their frequent opposition to leaders' proposals, nurses have struggled to express their own interpretation of their work and to assert their needs as workers on the job. Nurses' resistance to professionalization underscored the limitations of leaders' ideology and strategies. Leaders' efforts to improve nursing education often served to divide nurses, isolating a select elite from the general body. Set on advancing the occupation of nursing, they often overlooked pressing needs of the women who were practicing it. And in their attempts to secure nurses' positions in hospitals, they have supported the growth of a complex, rigid hierarchy for nursing and allied hospital fields.

Yet nurses' history also illustrates the limitations of informal resistance, whether in the culture of apprenticeship or in public-health nurses' brief control of a world apart. Private-duty nurses were too socially and physically isolated to pose a coherent alternative to leaders' strategies. Within the favorable conditions of the lay public-health movement, public-health nurses were able to build a separate work situation for themselves, but they could not defend it when those conditions changed. In hospitals, nurses used the resources of institutional employment to gain more control over their work, but they still lacked the satisfaction and security of clearly acknowledged and legitimated authority. If leaders lacked sensitivity to most nurses' needs, nurses on the job often lacked the resources and the organization to press for effective changes.

Despite their limitations, nursing leaders have left a legacy of resources that nurses could apply to revised goals. Their self-consciousness and identification with work have provided nurses with an ideology of entitlement to authority and a model for commitment to work. Although nursing superintendents and nurses on the job resisted the goals of professional leaders, their own work orientations and work cultures were often supported and strengthened by the history and social organizations that leaders had built. Nurses' work culture gained a special cohesiveness and continuity from its location within a highly self-conscious occupational group. Nurses come to their work groups and their workplaces with a common tradition. Manuals on nursing techniques and ethical problems and didactic novels by nurses offered models of appropriate behavior at work. Historical accounts of the profession emphasized the social significance of nursing. Journals provided nurses with a sense of common purpose and a forum for discussing shared problems. Professional associations gave nurses much of the apparatus for sustaining and perpetuating a strong occupational identity.

Moreover, professional ideology embodied values that led nurses beyond the role of "the physician's hand." Although many observers have seen nurses' supposed "professionalism" as a conservative force that leads nurses to identify themselves with doctors, managers, and employers, the professional goal of autonomy in work also offers a model for a worker-defined view of the job that may support challenges to medical and administrative control. If leaders could shake off the elitism and self-defeating deference to hierarchy that have characterized their struggle for professionalization—if, indeed, they could exchange that goal for a more generous and inclusive program—they and other nurses could turn the re-sources and energy of the nursing organizations toward the pursuit of expanded authority for all nurses.

Recent responses to the problems of hospital work indi-cate some of the directions that nurses are exploring, both individually and collectively. Some are leaving hospital set-tings altogether, seeking refuge in new forms of health-care delivery. Like the old public-health agencies, health mainte-nance organizations or satellite clinics give nurses more prom-inent roles in screening and advising patients, and nurses find that the bonds of medical hierarchy loosen outside the hospi-tal. Organizations like these are likely to become more and more common, for preventive care or treatment given outside the hospital provides welcome economies of scale and lower overhead in a time of steeply escalating costs. In some places, nurses have sought to extend their independence at work by setting up their own practices, following the traditional en-trepreneurial model of private medicine. Some state boards have organized and certified independent practice in nurse-practitioner programs, postgraduate training that licenses the nurse to take on extended duties and to exercise a limited authority to diagnose and prescribe, either within or outside a hospital setting.[4]

Choices like these have helped to redefine the legitimate sphere of nursing practice in state law, within hospital walls, and in communities where independent nurses work. Nurse-practitioners and nurses in nontraditional workplaces offer an important model of nurses' capacities and nursing's possibili-ties. But these new options will not in themselves resolve the larger dilemmas of nursing. First, it seems likely that hospitals will remain the primary workplaces for nurses, and that most nurses will locate themselves within a conventional hospital division of labor. Only a minority will have the time and opportunity to seek out the nurse-practitioner's special train-ing, or to find or create jobs outside hospitals at a time when those institutions are offering more and more incentives to lure skilled workers. Indeed, nurses are far more often choosing to improve on private-duty nurses' old prerogatives as freelancers. Especially in large cities, increasing numbers of nurses work with local employment agencies, or "medical pools," rather than attaching themselves to any one institution. The pools provide good benefits and send their nurses to well-paid temporary jobs; hospitals desperate to fill in sparse workforces create a favorable market for this arrangement. Second, hospital-based research and care will almost certainly continue to dominate medical science and practice. To win a secure authority for themselves, nurses must do more than the old public-health nurses, whose elitism separated them from other nurses even as their marginality removed them from medical dominance. Instead, they must claim recognition in the workplace at the social and cultural center of medicine, and they must insist on the value of the nurse with conventional training even as they seek to broaden postgraduate education and opportunities for all nurses.

Inside hospitals, nurses will undoubtedly continue to feel the pressure of heavy workloads and often conflicting responsibilities to doctors, administrators, and patients. Very likely they will extend their longstanding efforts to claim a measure of control over hospital policies, and they will continue to resist an employer-defined view of their work with their own nursing theory and practice. From the call to "total patient care" to the elaboration of the nurse's new role as "patient advocate," nurses have worked to define their relationships with patients as the center of their work and as their sphere of legitimate authority. But as hospital nurses well know, the call to bring nurses "back to the bedside" is not easily translated from rhetoric to reality. Every plan to revise nursing practice must ultimately confront the structural constraints imposed by hospital administration. Nurses simply cannot hope to give ideal care in overcrowded, under-staffed, poorly maintained workplaces. Proposals for "nursing autonomy" are doomed unless nurses link them to broader issues of hospital work. Good patient care requires adequate staffing, decent equipment, careful maintenance. To ensure those conditions and to gain real legitimacy for their own work, nurses will need more than informal authority. They will need a real voice in medical decisions and in hospital management—more control than can be achieved in informal maneuvering, in token committee positions, or in their own present positions as middle managers. They will need to challenge and rethink the entrenched hierarchies of hospital life and the divisions of gender, class, and race that they reflect. They will need to negotiate new relationships with both doctors and administrators, and to reexamine their own relationships with licensed practical nurses, nurses' aides, and orderlies.

Moreover, nurses will have to go beyond the limitations and flaws of the current effort to upgrade bedside nursing. The new career ladders represent a promising attempt to provide concrete rewards and incentives for good patient care. But movement up these ladders is still based on restrictive credentials, frequently tied to degree requirements. The professional associations are not likely to take the lead in making these new roles more accessible. Ordinary nurses must press both hospital administrators and their own leaders—not by fighting for a return to apprenticeship education, but by insisting on credit for their experience and by demanding access to continuing education through hospital or other institutional funding.

Finally, nurses will have to think long and hard about the broader implications of their new role as patient advocates. At its best, this role represents a strong humanitarian ideal, a commitment to support others at times of suffering and vulnerability. As large, profitable plants and as centers of scientific research, hospitals surely need these reminders of their social responsibility to the sick. But when nurses take on the role of patient advocate, will they do more than merely re-create and reinforce the sexual division of labor that assigns women to "caring" and male physicians to "curing"? We will do well to remember that "total patient care" was first elaborated in the 1950s, when nurses' authority was being attacked in popular culture and social science, and when the feminine mystique celebrated female domesticity over commitment to work. As patient advocates, will nurses fight for needed structural changes, or will they be content to act as the "heart" of the hospital while physicians and administrators remain at its head?

In efforts to gain more formal and secure prerogatives at work, increasing numbers of hospital nurses are turning to unionization as an alternative to the professional associations. Since the mid-1960s, a new wave of organization has brought more state nurses' associations (SNAs) into the business of collective bargaining, and as in the 1940s, nursing leaders have responded by taking a stronger position in favor of unionization. In the early 1970s, the ANA extended its commitment to the Economic Security Program by working actively to reclaim legal bargaining rights for nurses. In terms recalling the group's consistent commitment to "professional autonomy," the ANA president endorsed unionization. "By acting as a cohesive group, rather than as individual professionals, nurses will achieve the right to make decisions that affect them, their practice, and the quality of care." The organization lobbied to end the exemption of nonprofit hospitals from the obligations set out for employers in the National Labor Relations Act. In July 1974, the hospital exemption of Taft-Hartley was revoked, and nurses finally regained the legal right to collective bargaining.[5]

More state nurses' associations have been certified as bargaining units in a surge of organization since the mid-1960s. While some hospital unions have limited their demands to traditional bread-and-butter issues, SNAs have sought to respond to the problems nurses face on the hospital floor. In Chicago's Cook County Hospital, for example, striking nurses represented by the Illinois Nurses' Association refused administrators' efforts to pit them against patients, linking demands for better hours, limited overtime, and adequate break-time with protests about the quality of patient care under existing conditions. In two Rhode Island hospitals, nurses bargained for contracts that would guarantee appropriate nurse-patient ratios, simultaneously defending patient care and resisting the increasing pace of work. In these and other negotiations, nurses have fought for more say in decisions that affect nursing care. As one striking nurse explained, "I want to feel good about myself as a professional nurse, and the only way I can do that is to be sure the conditions under which I work are good enough for my patient."[6]

At the bargaining table and sometimes on the picket line, nurses have shown a determination and sense of common interests that belie stereotypes of their passivity as women and as doctors' subordinates. Renouncing the no-strike pledge and winning the legal right to bargain, nurses have begun to rewrite the old formula that equated "professionalism" with hostility to unions. Members of one successful professional association in Washington, D.C., proclaimed this new spirit on t-shirts that read, "A Nurse's Place Is in Her Union," buoyantly redefining their proper roles as women and as "professionals."

Old ties between nurses and the labor movement have been renewed over the last ten or fifteen years. In the 1960s, a wave of white-collar and public-sector unionism moved organized labor from its traditional strongholds in the declining industrial sector into the new workplaces of service occupations. Faced with its own waning strength and influence, organized labor began to look to these new and active constituencies. Perhaps, too, the activism of the civil rights movement and later the women's movement have helped to create greater social awareness of the claims and activities of groups that have long been underrepresented in the labor movement as in other institutions. Nurses themselves sometimes turned from SNAs to unions, again expressing a traditional dissatisfaction and impatience with the style and organization of the professional associations. Whether organized in professional associations or in unions, more nurses feel a sense of identity with the labor movement; and, in turn, more unions have grown attentive to nurses as workers and begun to recruit nurses and other hospital workers into their ranks.[7]

Nurses' work lives have always been informed by life

outside the workplace as well as by the immediate environment of the job, and hospital nursing is no exception. Nursing leaders and educators had drawn on the experience of their medical colleagues as a model of successful professionalization, and had shared the excitement and career commitment of the first generation of college women. Private-duty nurses demanded the work and social prerogatives of the "new woman," even as their own employment prospects deteriorated. Public-health nurses had allied themselves with the reform impulse and the organizations of the larger public-health movement. All had found sources of strength, even in a culture that was indifferent or hostile to women's work. In different ways, all had also run up against the marginality of their positions as women and as workers. Leaders never won professional autonomy and only slowly gained university status for nurses' education; private-duty nurses were squeezed out of a rationalized scheme of work; public-health nurses saw their self-organization absorbed into the institutions of mainstream medicine and nursing.

In facing many of the same structural obstacles, hospital nurses can turn to a revitalized women's movement. Influenced by the energy and renewed organization of the women's movement, nurses have begun to analyze their positions as women in a sex-segregated workforce. For some, feminism has stimulated a sense of the limitations of professional organization. In Pennsylvania, for example, members of Nurses Now, a task force of the National Organization for Women, have remained active in their SNA, but defended the need for a separate feminist organization: "Many feminist issues are so inbred in nursing that we believe we can argue them more effectively from a feminist view, rather than a solely professional one."[8] The resurgence of feminism has moved some nurses to challenge the basis of medical hierarchy and its rituals of deference. Most have abandoned the old forms of hospital etiquette, no longer standing up or moving aside to acknowledge the august presence of a doctor. And they are beginning to notice and reject the more subtle forms of hierarchy that pervade the doctor-nurse relationship.

The growth of white-collar unionism and the revival of the women's movement both have offered nurses new ideological and organizational support, resources that extend nurses' ability to challenge the limitations of their work. But the impetus for that struggle comes from nurses' own occupational traditions. In professional associations, in the enclosed worlds of nursing schools, and on the job, nurses have long set forth their own conceptions of themselves as women and as workers. Nurses today are reclaiming and defending the strengths of their history as "the physician's hand." As feminists they are refuting the portrayal of nurses as incomplete doctors or downtrodden adjuncts to insist on their extensive and indispensable contributions to the work of health care. At the same time, they continue to resist the traditional connotations of "the physician's hand," with all it has implied of passivity, self-abnegation, and subordination.

The strength and persistence of nursing's various work cultures qualify the dominant sociological and historical assessment of the meaning of women's experience as paid workers. Much recent study has argued that paid work simply mirrors and reinforces existing gender relationships. The argument goes that most women's work experience confirms the cultural message of female inferiority and subordination: they labor under the authority of male supervisors and employers; they work at jobs that may be considerably less appealing than traditional domestic duties and that carry little prestige, outlet for initiative, or possibility of advancement. Women earn too little to find real alternatives to marriage and family life through wage work, so most experience paid labor, not as a new departure, but rather as an extension of their place in the family.[9]

This interpretation is forceful and persuasive. But nursing history suggests that it is too static and one-dimensional to encompass the totality of working women's experience and consciousness. The structure of paid work undeniably replicates existing relationships of power and inequality: the stratification of the workforce clearly reproduces hierarchies organized by race, class, and gender. But for women, the expansion of paid work also held other, unanticipated, consequences and contradictory possibilities. When women moved into nursing as an occupation, they did not simply transfer nineteenth-century values of womanly service and feminine nurturing into a new setting, nor did they docilely exchange the authority of fathers or husbands in the home for that of male doctors in the hospital. Rather, nurses entered a realm that both confirmed and contradicted cultural expectations for women. Throughout their history, nurses were exposed to professional ideology through a small group of elite leaders, and they participated in a strong tradition of apprenticeship and initiation in nursing schools. Both experiences motivated sustained involvement in paid work, a socialization which subverted common expectations for female domesticity. As paid workers, nurses drew closer to a "male" public world. They took on some of the values and traditions of that world, even as they interpreted work through the lens of female experience and often reshaped it by drawing on available models for women outside the workplace. As well, the changing possibilities of work itself impelled nurses toward an altered perception of themselves as women. Over the twentieth century, the actual content of nursing work became increasingly anomalous for women: the technological and social mystique of modern medicine enhanced nurses' expertise and authority in ways that implicitly threatened traditional conceptions of women's work. And as hospital expansion increased the demand for nurses' services, they found in scarcity a new confirmation of their value on the job.

It may be that nurses constitute a kind of labor aristocracy among women; privileged in comparison to other female workers, perhaps nurses are exceptional. Yet by the same token, it may turn out that women in other occupations also develop a sense of pride and self-esteem in the daily context of their workplaces, through the informal exchanges of the workday, in the rituals of initiation that are part of most jobs.[10] Certainly other women, like nurses, have been drawn into the workforce as the expanding service sector creates new opportunities for paid work. And as more women spend more of their lives at wage-earning work, the cultural ideology dictating that woman's place is in the home will surely come under renewed pressures and challenges.

Until we know more about women in different occupations, until we move from a focus on the structure of work to an examination of women's experiences and consciousness, we cannot assume that the undeniable constraints of women's work have obliterated women's human capacity to discover the opportunities of changed circumstances and to use them to remake and transform their experience. Without losing sight of the institutional limits that bound women's work, we might yet begin to reassess the impact of work as we discover the record of women's resilience and resistance on the job. We might then confirm what nursing history powerfully suggests: that the experience of paid work does not merely reinforce women's subordination. Instead, work can heighten the contradictions that women confront as social actors who are both participants and outsiders in their own culture. The experience of paid work changes women's lives, sometimes in ways that challenge and disrupt existing notions of the place of women.

NOTES

INTRODUCTION

1. Florence Nightingale, *Notes on Nursing: What It Is, and What It Is Not* (New York: Appleton, 1860), p. 3.

2. Alfred Worcester, *Nurses and Nursing* (Cambridge; Mass.: Harvard Univ. Press, 1927), p. 9.

3. Phrase "twilight and darkness" from Elizabeth Marion Jamieson and Mary Sewall, *Trends in Nursing History: Their Relationship to World Events*, 2nd ed. (Philadelphia: W. B. Saunders, 1944; 1st ed., 1940), p. 295. Other major nursing histories include Mary Adelaide Nutting and Lavinia L. Dock, *A History of Nursing* (New York: Putnam, 1907–12); Mary M. Roberts, *American Nursing: History and Interpretation* (New York: Macmillan, 1954); Lucy Ridgeley Seymer, *A General History of Nursing*, 4th ed. (London: Faber and Faber, 1956; 1st ed., 1932); Lena Dixon Dietz, *History and Modern Nursing* (Philadelphia: F. A. Davis, 1963); Minnie Goodnow, *Nursing History*, 7th ed. (Philadelphia: W. B. Saunders, 1942; 1st ed., 1916). For two recent additions, see Lynda Flanagan, *One Strong Voice: The Story of the American Nurses' Association* (Kansas City, Mo.: The Lowell Press, 1964) and Gwendolyn Safier, *Contemporary American Leaders in Nursing: An Oral Account* (New York: McGraw-Hill, 1977).

4. "A Statement of Policy," *RN* 1 (Oct. 1937): 4; and *RN* 1 (May 1938): 9.

5. I developed this definition of work culture in close collaboration with Susan Porter Benson; see her article, " 'The Clerking Sisterhood': Rationalization and the Work Culture of Saleswomen in American Department Stores, 1890–1960," *Radical America* 12 (March–April 1978): 41–55. For other discussions of shopfloor culture, see David Montgomery, *Workers' Control in America* (Cambridge, England: Cambridge Univ. Press, 1979); Ken C. Kusterer, *Know-How on the Job: The Important Knowledge of "Unskilled" Workers* (Boulder, Colo.: Westview Replication Press, 1978); Monte A. Calvert, *The Mechanical Engineer in America, 1830–1910: Professional Cultures in Conflict* (Baltimore: Johns Hopkins University Press, 1967). Sociolinguists have offered stimulating theoretical and ethnographic descriptions. See John J. Gumperz and Dell Hymes, eds., *Directions in Sociolinguistics: The Ethnography of Experience* (New York: Holt, Rinehart and Winston, 1972), and Dell Hymes, ed., *Reinventing Anthropology* (New York: Random House, 1969). Medical sociologists have contributed a number of sensitive ethnographies; three classics with material on nursing are Rose Laub Coser, *Life in the Wards* (East Lansing, Mich.: Michigan State Univ. Press, 1962); Temple Burling, Edith M. Lentz, and Robert N.

Wilson, *The Give and Take in Hospitals* (New York: G. P. Putnam, 1956); and Leonard Reissman and John H. Rohrer, eds., *Change and Dilemma in the Nursing Profession* (New York: G. P. Putnam's Sons, 1957).

6. Much of this literature outlines the structural constraints of sex-segregation, and a related interpretive literature emphasizes the ways in which paid work reinforces women's oppression. Theoretical statements of this viewpoint include Juliet Mitchell, *Woman's Estate* (New York: Vintage, 1971); Margaret Benston, "The Political Economy of Women's Liberation," *Monthly Review* 21 (1969): 13–38; Paddy Quick, "Women's Work," *Review of Radical Political Economics*, summer 1972, pp. 2–19; Heidi Hartman, "Capitalism, Patriarchy, and Job Segregation by Sex," in Martha Blaxall and Barbara Reagan, eds., *Women and the Workplace: The Implications of Occupational Segregation* (Chicago: Univ. of Chicago Press, 1976), 137–69.

Historical interpretations that share this perspective include Louise A. Tilly and Joan W. Scott, *Women, Work, and Family* (New York: Holt, Rinehart, and Winston, 1978), and Leslie Woodcock Tentler, *Wage-Earning Women: Industrial Work and Family Life in the United States, 1900–1930* (New York: Oxford Univ. Press, 1979). For another view of the relationship between women's work and family life, see Alice Kessler-Harris, *Out to Work: A History of Wage-Earning Women in the United States* (New York: Oxford Univ. Press, 1982).

These studies apply the analysis to nursing in more detail: Eva Gamarnikow, "Sexual Division of Labour: The Case of Nursing," in Annette Kuhn and AnnMarie Wolpe, eds., *Feminism and Materialism: Women and Modes of Production* (London, Henley, Boston: Routledge and Kegan Paul, 1978), 96–123; and Jo Ann Ashley, *Hospitals, Paternalism, and the Role of the Nurse* (New York: Teachers College Press, 1976).

Finally, an emerging social history of nursing is redefining approaches to the subject, as seen in Celia Davies, ed., *Rewriting Nursing History* (London: Croom Helm, and Totowa, N.J.: Barnes and Noble, 1980), on British nurses; and Ellen Condliffe Lagemann, ed., *Nursing History: New Perspectives, New Possibilities* (New York: Teachers College Press, forthcoming).

7. For discussions of pre-industrial work and the coming of industrial capitalism, see: Herbert Gutman, *Work, Culture, and Society in Industrializing America* (New York: Alfred A. Knopf, 1976); Milton Cantor, ed., *American Workingclass Culture* (Westport, Ct.: Greenwood, 1979); Alan Dawley, *Class and Community: The Industrial Revolution in Lynn* (Cambridge, Mass.: Harvard Univ. Press, 1976); Susan E. Hirsch, *Roots of the American Working Class: The Industrialization of Crafts in Newark, 1800–1860* (Philadelphia: Univ. of Pennsylvania Press, 1978); Bruce Laurie, *Working People of Philadelphia, 1800–1850* (Philadelphia: Temple Univ. Press, 1980). Twentieth-century interpretations of rationalization include Montgomery, *Workers' Control*; Daniel Nelson, *Managers and Workers: Origins of the New Factory System in the United States, 1880–1920* (Madison: Univ. of Wisconsin Press,

1975); and Harry Braverman, *Labor and Monopoly Capital: The Degradation of Work in the Twentieth Century* (New York: Monthly Review Press, 1974).

8. Notable exceptions include Benson, " 'The Clerking Sisterhood' "; Susan Reverby, "The Search for the Hospital Yardstick: Nursing and the Rationalization of Hospital Work," in Susan Reverby and David Rosner, eds., *Health Care in America* (Philadelphia: Temple Univ. Press, 1979); David Wagner, "The Proletarianization of Nursing in the United States, 1932–1946," *International Journal of Health Services* 10 (1980): 271–90; and Barbara Garson, *All the Live-long Day: The Meaning and Demeaning of Routine Work* (New York: Doubleday, 1975).

9. For the history of black nurses, see Adah B. Thoms, *Pathfinders* (New York: Kay, 1929), and Mabel Keaton Staupers, *No Time for Prejudice* (New York: Macmillan, 1961). New work on the subject includes Patricia E. Sloan, "Black Hospitals and Nurse Training Schools: The Formative Years, 1880–1900," and Darlene Clark Hine, "Mabel Keaton Staupers and Black Women Nurses: Integration of Black Nurses into the Armed Forces during World War II," papers presented at the Fifth Berkshire Conference on the History of Women, June 1981.

CHAPTER 1

1. For classic statements of this interpretation, see William J. Goode, "Community within a Community: The Professions," *American Sociological Review* 22 (April 1957): 194–200; Ernest Greenwood, "Attributes of a Profession," *Social Work* 2 (July 1957): 45–55; and Goode, "Encroachment, Charlatanism, and the Emerging Profession: Psychology, Medicine, and Sociology," *American Sociological Review* 25 (1960): 902–14. Other examples include Howard M. Vollmer and Donald L. Mills, eds., *Professionalization* (Englewood Cliffs, N.J.: Prentice-Hall, 1966); Wilbert E. Moore, *The Professions: Roles and Rules* (New York: Russell Sage, 1970); Amitai Etzioni, ed., *The Semi-Professions and Their Organization* (New York: The Free Press, 1969). For a summary of the literature with a more detailed categorization than the one offered here, see Jack Ladinsky, "The Professions," in Albert J. Wertheimer and Mickey C. Smith, eds., *Pharmacy Practice: Social and Behavioral Aspects*, 2nd ed. (Baltimore, Md.: University Park Press, 1981), pp. 1–11.

2. Julius A. Roth, "Professionalism: The Sociologist's Decoy," *Sociology of Work and Occupations* 1 (Feb. 1974): 6–23. See also J. A. Jackson, ed., *Professions and Professionalization* (Cambridge, England: Cambridge Univ. Press, 1970).

3. Eliot Freidson, *Profession of Medicine* (New York: Harper and Row, 1970).

4. For revisionist historical interpretations of medical professionalization, see Gerald E. Markowitz and David K. Rosner, "Doctors in Crisis: A Study in the Use of Medical Educational Reform to Establish Modern Professional Elitism in Medicine," *American Quarterly* 25 (March 1973): 83–107, and E. Richard Brown, *Rockefeller Medicine Men: Medicine and Capitalism in America* (Berkeley: Univ. of California Press, 1979).

5. For a related discussion of service orientation and professional ideology, see Harold L. Wilensky, "The Professionalization of Everyone?" *American Journal of Sociology* 80 (Sept. 1964): 137–58. For a revisionist interpretation that stresses the process of professionalization, see Douglas Klegon, "The Sociology of Professions: An Emerging Perspective," *Sociology of Work and Occupations* 5 (Aug. 1978): 259–83. A classic sociological analysis of the occupational culture of the professions is Everett Cherrington Hughes, *Men and Their Work* (Glencoe, Ill.: The Free Press, 1958).

6. For another discussion of gender and work in nursing see Eva Gamarnikow, "Sexual Division of Labour: The Case of Nursing," in Annette Kuhn and AnnMarie Wolpe, eds., *Feminism and Materialism: Women and Modes of Production* (London, Henley, Boston: Routledge and Kegan Paul, 1978), pp. 96–123, and Jo Ann Ashley, *Hospitals, Paternalism, and the Role of the Nurse* (New York: Teachers College Press, 1976).

7. M. Victoria Pearson, "The Unrecognized Queen," *Trained Nurse and Hospital Review* (hereafter cited as *TNHR*) 64 (May 1920): 417.

8. Annie M. Brainard, *The Evolution of Public Health Nursing* (Philadelphia: W. B. Saunders, 1922), p. 420.

9. For cultural histories of work and professionalization, see Burton J. Bledstein, *The Culture of Professionalism: The Middle Class and the Development of Higher Education in America* (New York: W. W. Norton, 1976); Daniel T. Rodgers, *The Work Ethic in Industrial America, 1850–1920* (Chicago: Univ. of Chicago Press, 1978); and Robert Wiebe, *The Search for Order, 1877–1920* (New York: Hill and Wang, 1967).

10. Frances M. Ott, "Private Duty, Past and Present, The Progress of Forty Years," *TNHR* 80 (June 1928): 696–99.

11. Gertrude C. Quigley, "Attitude in Bedside Nursing," *TNHR* 97 (Oct. 1936): 326–327.

12. Sister Rose Alexius, "The Heart of the Hospital, Expressing the Christlike Spirit," *TNHR* 71 (Dec. 1923): 518.

13. "Has the Nursing Instinct Died Out?" *TNHR* 73 (Nov. 1924): 438–39; "Is Religion in Our Schools Being Relinquished?" *TNHR* 76 (Jan. 1926): 38–39.

14. Letter from "A Pioneer Nurse," *TNHR* 65 (July 1920): 54–55; see also "Private Duty Problems," *TNHR* 73 (July 1924): 57–58; and Amy Armour Smith, "Getting Down to Brass Tacks a Model Budget for Private Duty Nurses," *TNHR* 74 (Jan. 1925), 25–29.

15. Letter from E.L.C., Ken., *American Journal of Nursing* (hereafter

cited as *AJN*) 22 (Dec. 1921): 208; letter from E.G.M., Mass., *AJN* 22 (Jan. 1922): 297–99; letter from M.M.G., Mo. and editor's note, *AJN* 22 (July 1922): 841–42.

16. "When Is Humor Humor?" *TNHR* 72 (April 1924): 366.

17. Mary E. Gladwin, *Ethics—Talks to Nurses* (Philadelphia: W. B. Saunders, 1930),p. 30.

18. Frances J. Patton, "Aspects of Private Duty Nursing in the South," *AJN* 20 (July 1920): 806–7.

19. Letter from "A Nurse Member," *Public Health Nursing* 16 (Jan. 1924): 2.

20. For an account of the patient's experience of nineteenth-century hospitals, see Charles Rosenberg, "And Heal the Sick: The Hospital and the Patient in Nineteenth-Century America," *Journal of Social History* 10 (summer 1977): 428–47. Many sources describe Nightingale's famous reforms; a typical account may be found in Elizabeth Marion Jamieson and Mary Sewall, *Trends in Nursing History: Their Relationship to World Events*, 2nd ed. (Philadelphia: W. B. Saunders, 1944; 1st ed.,1940), pp. 373–99. An invaluable source for the structural development of nursing and its status in the 1920s is May Ayres Burgess's rich survey, *Nurses, Patients, and Pocketbooks: Report of a Study of the Economics of Nursing* (New York: Committee on the Grading of Nursing Schools, 1928).

21. Linda Richards, *Reminiscences of Linda Richards, America's First Trained Nurse* (Boston: Whitcomb and Barrows, 1911), p. 63.

22. Elizabeth Christophers Hobson, *Recollections of a Happy Life* (New York: G. P. Putnam's Sons, 1916), p. 102.

23. Mary Roberts Rinehart, *My Story* (New York: Farrar and Rinehart, 1931), p. 47.

24. "Education and Intelligence: More Facts from the Grading Committee," *AJN* 28 (Sept. 1928): 910–11.

25. For accounts of the changing context of nineteenth-century medical practice, see Paul Starr, "Medicine, Economy and Society in Nineteenth-Century America," *Journal of Social History* 10 (summer 1977): 588–607; and Charles E. Rosenberg and Morris Vogel, eds., *The Therapeutic Revolution* (Philadelphia: Univ. of Pennsylvania Press, 1979). Morris J. Vogel describes changing patterns of hospital use in "The Transformation of the American Hospital, 1850–1920," in Susan Reverby and David Rosner, eds., *Health Care in America* (Philadelphia: Temple Univ. Press, 1979), pp. 105–16.

26. E. H. L. Corwin, *The American Hospital* (New York: The Commonwealth Fund, 1946), is an early history of institutional development. Recent histories of hospital care offer varied interpretations of the changing patterns of hospital use and the evolving mission of the hospital. In interpreting the move of medical care from patients' homes to doctors' offices and hospitals, Paul Starr considers the influence of a growing consumer

demand for medical services. David Rosner argues that the rising cost of new technology contributed to the shift in hospital funding from charitable sources to patients' fees: see "Business at the Bedside: Health Care in Brooklyn, 1890–1915," in Reverby and Rosner, *Health Care in America*, pp. 117–31. In *The Invention of the Modern Hospital, Boston, 1870–1930* (Chicago: Univ. of Chicago Press, 1980), Morris Vogel weighs the social and technological influences on increasing hospital use, emphasizing the impact of urbanization and changing family patterns. Stanley Joel Reiser's *Medicine and the Reign of Technology* (Cambridge, England: Cambridge Univ. Press, 1978) traces the development of medical technology and its role in transforming hospitals from caretaking institutions to centers for intensive treatment and medical research.

27. See Susan Reverby, "The Search for the Hospital Yardstick: Nursing and the Rationalization of Hospital Work," in Reverby and Rosner, *Health Care in America*, pp. 206–19; Reiser, *Medicine*, p. 152; Burgess, *Nurses, Patients*, p. 35; and Corwin, *American Hospital*, pp. 6–8. For more detailed accounts of early nursing schools with somewhat different interpretations, see Janet Wilson James, "Isabel Hampton and the Professionalization of Nursing in the 1890s," in Rosenberg and Vogel, *Therapeutic Revolution*, pp. 201–44; Nancy Tomes, " 'Little World of Our Own': The Pennsylvania Hospital Training School for Nurses, 1895–1907," *Journal of the History of Medicine and Allied Sciences* 33 (Oct. 1978): 507–30; and Jane E. Mottus, *New York Nightingales: The Emergence of the Nursing Profession at Bellevue and New York Hospital, 1850–1920* (Ann Arbor: University Microfilms International Research Press, 1981).

28. See, for example, editorial comment, "Some Common Obstacles to Progress," *AJN* 11 (March 1911): 420–22; and editorial comment, "The Nurse Pharisee," *AJN* 11 (April 1911): 503–4.

29. For a standard account of early professional associations and their restrictive membership, see Jamieson and Sewall, *Trends in Nursing History*, p. 464.

CHAPTER 2

1. "New Records," *RN* 35 (April 1972): 5, 7; "Who Works Where at What?" *RN* 37 (June 1974): 42.

2. Elizabeth Marion Jamieson and Mary Sewall, *Trends in Nursing History: Their Relationship to World Events*, 2nd ed. (Philadelphia: W. B. Saunders, 1944; 1st ed., 1940), p. 469; Minnie Goodnow, *Nursing History*, 7th ed. (Philadelphia: W. B. Saunders, 1942; 1st ed., 1916), p. 243. For recent interpretations, see Susan Armeny, "Resistance to Professionalization by American Trained Nurses, 1890–1905," paper presented at the

Fourth Berkshire Conference on the History of Women, Aug. 1978; and Nancy J. Tomes, "The Silent Battle: Registration in New York State, 1903–1920," in Ellen Condliffe Lagemann, ed., *Nursing History: New Perspectives, New Possibilities* (New York: Teachers College Press, forthcoming).

3. May Ayres Burgess, *Nurses, Patients, and Pocketbooks: Report of a Study of the Economics of Nursing* (New York: Committee on the Grading of Nursing Schools, 1928),p. 36.

4. Mary Adelaide Nutting, *Educational Status of Nursing*, U.S. Bureau of Education, Bull. 7, No. 475 (Washington, D.C.: G.P.O., 1912), p. 17.

5. Burgess, *Nurses, Patients*, pp. 35–37.

6. Beulah Crawford, "How and What to Teach in Nursing Ethics," *American Journal of Nursing* (hereafter cited as *AJN*) 26 (May 1926): 215.

7. Letter from "A Superintendent," *Trained Nurse and Hospital Review* (hereafter cited as *TNHR*) 85 (July 1930): 60.

8. Burgess, *Nurses, Patients*, p. 440.

9. Janet Wilson James makes the same suggestion; see her "Isabel Hampton and the Professionalization of Nursing in the 1890s," in Charles E. Rosenberg and Morris Vogel, eds., *The Therapeutic Revolution* (Philadelphia: Univ. of Pennsylvania Press, 1979), p. 235. For detailed data of nursing students' backgrounds, some of which suggests a slight decline in status after 1890, see Jane E. Mottus, *New York Nightingales: The Emergence of the Nursing Profession at Bellevue and New York Hospital, 1850–1920* (Ann Arbor: University Microfilms International Research Press, 1981), pp. 93–112.

10. "Education and Intelligence: More Facts from the Grading Committee," *AJN* 28 (Sept. 1928): 910–11.

11. Ibid. High school graduation increased rapidly through the 1920s and 1930s; in 1930, 68 percent of student nurses had high school diplomas. See *AJN* 30 (May 1930): 618–19.

12. Burgess, *Nurses, Patients*, pp. 241–42.

13. "State Registration Requirements for Entrance to Nursing Schools," *AJN* 30 (May 1930): 618–19; May Ayres Burgess and William Darrach, *Nursing Schools—Today and Tomorrow: Final Report of the Committee on the Grading of Nursing Schools* (New York, 1934), pp. 157–58.

14. Ella A. Taylor, "Allowances *versus* Tuition," *AJN* 35 (Oct. 1935): 971–72; "Allowances vs. Tuition in 1939," *AJN* 40 (Aug. 1940): 909–11.

15. Ella A. Taylor, "How Many Hours Are Students Working?" *AJN* 36 (Jan. 1936): 79–83.

16. See, for example, Ann Blumenthal, "An Outlined System for Moving Accepted Students through the Required Course of Training," *AJN* 30 (Jan. 1930): 75–80; "A Year's Survey of Ward Teaching," *AJN* 32 (April 1932): 445–51; Isabel M. Stewart, "What Educational Philosophy Shall We Accept for the New Curriculum?" *AJN* 35 (March 1935): 259–67.

17. Burgess and Darrach, *Nursing Schools*, pp. 147, 201; "Not Our School?" *AJN* 29 (Jan. 1929): 64.

18. Nursing Information Bureau, *Facts about Nursing* (New York: American Nurses' Association, 1942), p. 17.

19. "U.S. Cadet Nurse Corps," *TNHR* 111 (Sept. 1943): 202–3; *The U.S. Cadet Nurse Corps, 1943–1948* (Public Health Publication no. 38; Washington, D.C.: G.P.O., 1950); Mary M. Roberts, *American Nursing: History and Interpretation* (New York: Macmillan, 1954), pp. 385–90; Philip A. Kalisch and Beatrice J. Kalisch, *The Advance of American Nursing* (Boston: Little, Brown, 1978), pp. 473–75.

20. "College Field Program," *AJN* 44 (Feb. 1944): 175; "NNCWS [National Nursing Council for War Service] Plans Fall College Counseling Program," *AJN* 44 (Sept. 1944): 888; "College Counseling Program," *AJN* 44 (Oct. 1944): 994.

21. Esther Lucile Brown, *Nursing for the Future* (New York: Russell Sage, 1948), and National Nursing Council (NNC), *A Thousand Think Together* (New York, 1948). See especially Brown, p. 159 and NNC, p. 129.

22. Brown, *Nursing for the Future*, p. 49.

23. Helen Nahm, "Nursing Education Today—Its Advantages," *Nursing World* 127 (Aug. 1953): 18.

24. Isabel Hampton Robb, *Nursing Ethics for Hospital and Private Use* (Cleveland: Koeckert, 1928; first published in 1900), p. 50.

25. Caroline Duer, "Not Quite Nonsense about Nursing," *AJN* 46 (Oct. 1946): 680.

26. Cava Wilson, "Character," *AJN* 30 (March 1930): 278. See also Charlotte Aikens, *Studies in Ethics for Nurses* (Philadelphia: W. B. Saunders, 1923), p. 189.

27. Erving Goffman, *Asylums: Essays on the Social Situation of Mental Patients and Other Inmates* (Garden City, N.Y.: Doubleday-Anchor, 1961), pp. 3–12.

28. Interview with Sarah I., 12 March 1977; interview with Ruth I., 25 Oct. 1976.

Oral history provided an important source for the argument in this chapter. I sought to record nurses' memoirs to discover how ordinary nurses themselves experienced and interpreted their work. I did eleven interviews during 1976–77 and two more in 1979–80. The interviews were open-ended, although I asked all of the nurses similar questions to draw out their experiences in nursing school and later work. The taped records ranged from 45 minutes to three hours. I also used two transcripts of interviews in oral history collections, one done by the Bridgeport, Connecticut, Federal Writers Project and another from the University of Rhode Island's growing collection. My principles of selection were few: I looked for nurses who had trained in different regions at different times, I interviewed women who had graduated from nursing school before 1960 (except one), and I chose not to seek out women who were identified as professional leaders, as these women's experiences and perspectives are well documented elsewhere. The nurses in my sample were all female. Two of the fifteen were black women. Two had college degrees, while the rest came from hospital-based programs. Judging by the size of the hospitals, the programs and affiliations offered, and other sources of information about the particular schools, I would say that most of their alma maters were average or above average by the prevailing standards of their time. Their job histories covered a range. Most had spent most of their working lives in hospital jobs, reflecting the dominance of hospital-based practice since the 1940s. Two were administrators; two more had done extensive work in supervisory or administrative positions. One was a public-health nurse; another had done many years of private-duty work.

29. Interview with Astrid N., 23 Oct. 1976.

30. Caroline Hedger, M.D., "Health and the Student Nurse: Increasing Effectiveness during Training," *TNHR* 71 (Dec. 1923): 526–32.

31. Robb, *Nursing Ethics*, p. 173.

32. Interview with Emma F., 28 Oct. 1976; interview with Sarah I., 12 March 1977.

33. Louise Logan, *Nurse* (New York: Arcadia House, 1940), p. 46; on ritual mortification, see Goffman, *Asylums*, p. 23.

34. Logan, *Nurse*, p. 46.

35. Ann Forrest, *Yes, Doctor!* (Siloam Springs, Ark.: Bar D Press, 1939), p. 9.

36. Josephine Goldmark, *Nursing and Nursing Education in the United States: A Report of the Committee for the Study of Nursing Education* (New York: Macmillan, 1923), p. 228; Burgess and Darrach, *Nursing Schools*, p. 164.

37. Willie Carhart Morehead, *The Saving Grace* (New York: Vantage, 1953), p. 3.

38. Brunettie Burrow, *Angels in White* (San Antonio, Tex.: Naylor, 1959), p. 3.

39. Mary Roberts Rinehart, *My Story* (New York: Farrar and Rinehart, 1931), p. 53.

40. Agnes Gelinas, *Nursing and Nursing Education* (New York: The Commonwealth Fund, 1946), pp. 39–40; Brown, *Nursing for the Future*, pp. 48, 164.

41. Helen Dore Boylston, *Sue Barton, Student Nurse* (Boston: Little, Brown, 1936), p. 23. Boylston was a nurse as well as the author of this popular series.

42. Sara E. Parsons, *Nursing Problems and Obligations* (Boston: Whitcomb and Barrows, 1916), p. 39.

43. Robb, *Nursing Ethics*, p. 73.

44. See Mary Douglas, *Purity and Danger* (London: Routledge and Kegan Paul, 1966), for an anthropological interpretation of the meaning and uses of cultural taboos that develop around biological processes.

45. Mary E. Gladwin, *Ethics—Talks to Nurses* (Philadelphia: W. B. Saunders, 1930), p. 97.

46. Interview with Anna D., 25 Oct. 1976.

47. Eugenia Kennedy Spalding, *Professional Adjustments in Nursing for Senior Students and Graduates* (Philadelphia: Lippincott, 1939), p. 379.

48. Parsons, *Nursing Problems*, p. 39.

49. Alice L. Price, "Prelude to Duty: Interpreting the Rhythm of Ward Service," *TNHR* 105 (Nov. 1940): 380.

50. Interview with Sarah I., 12 March 1977.

51. Interview with Rebecca T., 15 March 1977.

52. Corinne Johnson Kern, *I Go Nursing* (New York: E. P. Dutton, 1933), pp. 21–24.

53. Burrow, *Angels*, pp. 14, 80.

54. Rinehart, *My Story*, p. 75. Well known for her intrepid nurse-detective Miss Pinkerton, Rinehart herself was a nurse.

55. Interview with Alice S., 26 Oct. 1976.

56. Interview with Anna D., 25 Oct. 1976.

57. John E. Showalter, "Pediatric Nurses Dream of Death," in Ann M. Earle, Nina T. Argondizzo, and Austin H. Kutscher, eds., *The Nurse as Caregiver for the Terminal Patient and His Family* (New York: Columbia University Press, 1976), pp. 147–59.

58. See, for example, Doctor X, *Intern* (New York: Harper and Row, 1965), and the autobiographical novel, Samuel Shem, M.D. *The House of God* (New York: Dell, 1981). Another intriguing example is Elizabeth Morgan, *The Making of a Woman Surgeon* (New York: G. P. Putnam, 1980); Morgan's self-conscious concerns about femininity make a jarring contrast to her story of initiation into the surgeon's code of decisive and unemotional demeanor.

59. See, for example, Ella Rothweiler, John S. Coulter, and Felix Jansey, *The Science and Art of Nursing* (Philadelphia: F. A. Davis, 1936), pp. 96–97; Parsons, *Nursing Problems*, p. 52; Aikens, *Studies in Ethics for Nurses*, pp. 51, 143–44.

60. Gertrude E. Mallette, *Into the Wind* (Garden City, N.Y.: Doubleday, 1941), p. 77.

61. Corinne Johnson Kern, *I Was a Probationer* (New York: E. P. Dutton, 1937), p. 119.

62. Robb, *Nursing Ethics*, p. 216.

62. Mary Sewall Gardner, *Katharine Kent* (New York: Macmillan, 1946), p. 69.

64. Aikens, *Studies in Ethics for Nurses*, p. 51.

65. Parsons, *Nursing Problems*, p. 52.

66. Rothweiler, Coulter, and Jansey, *Science and Art of Nursing*, p. 96.

67. Mae Francis Colby, "Not in the Archives: True Stories by a Private Duty Nurse," *TNHR* 107 (Sept. 1941): 199.

68. Mallette, *Into the Wind*, pp. 72–73.

69. Ibid., p. 256.

70. Kern, *Probationer*, pp. 136, 150–51.

71. Ibid., pp. 221, 298.

72. Boylston, *Sue Barton, Student Nurse*, p. 218, 243.

73. Helen Wells, *Cherry Ames, Senior Nurse* (New York: Grosset and Dunlap, 1944), p. 107.

74. Dora E. Birchard, "The Birth of a Nurse," *TNHR* 94 (Feb. 1935): 161–62.

75. Blanche Poulter, "A Cadet Gets Her Cap," *TNHR* 113 (Aug. 1944): 100.

76. These examples are from *RN*, "Calling All Nurses"; see: vol. 1, Jan. 1938, p. 30; Aug. 1938, p. 33; vol. 2, Nov. 1938, p. 30; Dec. 1938, p. 37; Feb. 1939, p. 29; May 1939, p. 29.

77. For a discussion of nineteenth-century women's culture, see Carroll Smith-Rosenberg, "The Female World of Love and Ritual: Relations between Women in Nineteenth-Century America," *Signs* 1 (autumn 1975): 1–29; for the influence of close female friendships in women's colleges and female reform, see Nancy Sahli, "Smashing: Women's Relationships before the Fall," *Chrysalis* 8 (1979): 17–27; and Blanche Wiesen Cook, "Female Support Networks and Political Activism: Lillian Wald, Crystal Eastman, and Emma Goldman," *Chrysalis* 3 (1977): 43–61. For work on the changing character of social life in the twentieth century, see Christina Simmons, "Companionate Marriage and the Lesbian Threat," *Frontiers* 4 (Fall 1979): 54–59, and Simmons, " 'Marriage in the Modern Manner': Sexual Radicalism and Reform in America, 1914–41" (Ph.D. diss. Brown University, 1982). For a survey of women's relationships and an interpretation of the shifting context of the twentieth century, see Lillian Faderman, *Surpassing the Love of Men: Romantic Friendship and Love between Women from the Renaissance to the Present* (New York: William Morrow and Company, 1981).

78. Robb, *Nursing Ethics*, pp. 63–64, 139–40.

79. Rothweiler, Coulter, and Jansey, *Science and Art of Nursing*, p. 95.

80. Camilla A. Anderson, *Emotional Hygiene: The Art of Understanding* (Philadelphia: Lippincott, 1943), p. 142.

81. Mary Williams Brinton, *My Cap and My Cape* (Philadelphia: Dorrance, 1950), p. 16.

82. Parsons, *Nursing Problems*, p. 67; see also Gladwin, *Ethics*, pp. 186–87; Lena Dixon Dietz, *Professional Problems of Nurses*, 2nd ed. (Phil-

adelphia: F. A. Davis, 1936), p. 125; and Gardner, *Katharine Kent*, pp. 18–19.

83. Helen Dore Boylston, *Sue Barton, Visiting Nurse* (Boston: Little, Brown, 1938), p. 9; see also Wells, *Cherry Ames, Senior Nurse*, p. 200.

84. "The Refresher Student Speaks," *AJN* 41 (Dec. 1941): 1417.

85. "Marriage—Patriotism—Nursing," *AJN* 42 (Sept. 1942): 1048–49.

86. Interview with Anna D., 25 Oct. 1976.

87. "What Will You Do?" *TNHR* 107 (Nov. 1941): 367.

88. Janet M. Geister, "More Plain Talk," *TNHR* 108 (Jan. 1942): 198.

89. Letter from "Retired Nurse," *TNHR* 108 (Jan. 1942): 37.

90. Letter from R.N., New York, *AJN* 49 (June 1949): 4-adv.

91. Letter from Mary R. Walcher, R.N., Fargo, N.D., *RN* 13 (Nov. 1949): 14, 16.

92. Edith F. M. Pritchard, "Inherent Nursing Values vs. Professional Snobbery," *TNHR* 120 (June 1948): 419–20. See also Winifred Robin Clarke, R.N., "In Defense of the Hospital School of Nursing," *RN* 13 (May 1950): 28, 64.

93. Elizabeth C. Payne, R.N., B.S., "Who Should Be a Nurse?" *RN* 12 (July 1949): 32.

94. Letter from Effie L. McMichael, R.N., Oklahoma City, Okla., *RN* 16 (Sept. 1953): 14, 17.

95. Dana Hudson, "Nursing Education Today—Its Disadvantages," *Nursing World* 127 (Aug. 1953): 19; Franceska Rich, "Authoritarianism in Nursing," *RN* 17 (Oct. 1954): 44, 47, 74; letter from Genevieve M. Renstrom, R.N., Ill., *AJN* 49 (Oct. 1949): 6-adv.; Marjorie T. Henry, R.N., "Quantity or Quality?" *RN* 15 (April 1952): 39–40, 57, 59.

96. See Burgess, *Nurses, Patients*, pp. 51, 245, 250, 251.

97. Nursing Information Bureau, *Facts about Nursing* (New York: American Nurses' Association, 1950), pp. 13–14.

98. For a more detailed discussion and interpretation, see Barbara Melosh, "Doctors, Patients, and 'Big Nurse': Work and Gender in the Postwar Hospital," in Ellen Condliffe Lagemann, ed., *Nursing History: New Perspectives, New Possibilities* (New York: Teachers College Press, forthcoming).

99. Kalisch and Kalisch, *Advance of American Nursing*, pp. 510–11, 517–18; Karl R. Schneck, "The Nurse—BS or RN?" *Hospital Management* 69 (Jan. 1950): 29–31; "Looking Forward: Classification Clamor," *Modern Hospital* 74 (Feb. 1950): 41. The NOHSN later conducted its own survey of diploma programs, reported in Fred Couey and Elizabeth D. Couey, *Improving the Hospital School of Nursing* (Georgia State College of Business Administration, 1957).

100. "Shorter Training?" *RN* 10 (May 1947): 49.

101. Described in "*RN* Speaks: Compromise or Conversion?" *RN* 12 (Nov. 1948): 30–31, 64, 66, 68, 71–72.

102. Schneck, "The Nurse—BS or RN?" p. 30.

103. Eli Ginzberg, *A Program for the Nursing Profession* (New York: Macmillan, 1948), p. 54.

104. "MD Scores Nursing's Bid for Professional Status," *RN* News, *RN* 26 (Jan. 1963): 21–22.

105. See Kalisch and Kalisch, *Advance of American Nursing*, pp. 515–18; and contemporary discussions, for example: "AMA Opposes Federal Aid to Student Nurses," *RN* 27 (Aug. 1964): 25–26; "AMA Opposes ANA's Salary/Education Goals," *RN* 30 (Jan. 1967): 24.

106. Interview with Anna D., 25 Oct. 1976; interviews with Astrid N., 23 Oct. 1976 and 25 Oct. 1976.

107. Letter from E.E., Connecticut R.N., *AJN* 38 (Jan. 1938): 93.

108. Interview with Lorraine S., 26 Oct. 1976.

109. Lavinia Dock, letter to hospital superintendents, *National Hospital Record*, Jan. 15, 1909, quoted in Nutting, *Educational Status*, p. 27.

CHAPTER 3

1. May Ayres Burgess, *Nurses, Patients, and Pocketbooks: Report of a Study of the Economics of Nursing* (New York: Committee on the Grading of Nursing Schools, 1928), pp. 197–202, 340; *American Journal of Nursing* (hereafter cited as ASN) 27 (July 1927): 518.

2. See, for example, David Montgomery, *Workers' Control in America* (Cambridge, England: Cambridge Univ. Press, 1979), and other works cited in introduction, note 7.

3. Burgess, *Nurses, Patients*, pp. 77, 98.

4. Genevieve E. Kidd, "Professional Obligations of Private Duty Nurses," *AJN* 20 (Jan. 1920): 290.

5. Interview with M. P., 30 April 1978; this informant was from an upper middle-class family that frequently employed private-duty nurses in the 1920s.

6. Quoted in Burgess, *Nurses, Patients*, p. 320.

7. Ibid., pp. 98, 102, 104, 105, 326, 338, 362; *Trained Nurse and Hospital Review* (hereafter cited as *TNHR*) 73 (Nov. 1924): 444; letter from M. E., Washington, *AJN* 28 (Aug. 1928): 831; letter from "A Married Nurse," *AJN* 28 (Oct. 1928): 1046.

8. Manuals discussed the special problems of "professional etiquette" in the isolated situation of private duty; see Isabel Hampton Robb, *Nursing Ethics for Hospital and Private Use* (Cleveland: Koeckert, 1928; first published in 1900), pp. 251, 257; Sara E. Parsons, *Nursing Problems and Obligations*

(Boston: Whitcomb and Barrows, 1916), p. 58; and Mary Louise Habel and Hazel Doris Milton, *The Graduate Nurse in the Home* (Philadelphia: Lippincott, 1939), pp. 37, 122–23. For discussions of ethical problems in specific private-duty cases, see examples in *TNHR* 73 (Aug, 1925): 147; *TNHR* 70 (Feb. 1923): 158; and *TNHR* 84 (Feb. 1930): 229.

9. Robb, *Nursing Ethics*, p. 197.

10. Both examples in "Oh Wad the Power Gie Us to See Ourselves as Ithers See Us," *TNHR* 79 (Aug. 1927): 147–50.

11. Parsons, *Nursing Problems*, p. 21; Habel and Milton, *The Graduate Nurse*, p. 184; letter from E. S. M., "Why One Family Was Glad When the Nurse Left," *AJN* 23 (Feb. 1923): 418–19. See also "The Trained Nurse—a Plea and a Protest," *AJN* 24 (Oct. 1924): 1025–28.

12. Quoted in Burgess, *Nurses, Patients*, p. 225; quoted in Walter B. Jones and R. E. Iffert, *Fitness for Nursing: A Study of Student Selection in Schools of Nursing* (Pittsburgh, Pa.: Bureau of Educational Records and Research, 1933), p. 12; Helen Wells, *Cherry Ames, Private Duty Nurse* (New York: Grosset and Dunlap, 1946), p. 147; and Mary E. Gladwin, *Ethics— Talks to Nurses* (Philadelphia: W. B. Saunders, 1930), p. 103.

13. Letter from R.N., Chicago, Ill., *RN* 2 (Dec. 1938): 4.

14. Gladwin, *Ethics*, p. 103. See also Ella Rothweiler, John S. Coulter, and Felix Jansey, *The Science and Art of Nursing* (Philadelphia: F. A. Davis, 1936), pp. 90–91; Charlotte Aikens, *Studies in Ethics for Nurses* (Philadelphia: W. B. Saunders, 1923), pp. 277–78; May Ayres Burgess and William Darrach, *Nursing Schools—Today and Tomorrow: Final Report of the Committee on the Grading of Nursing Schools* (New York, 1932), p. 69; and Lora Wood Hughes, *No Time for Tears* (Boston: Houghton-Mifflin, 1946), pp. 265–67.

15. Hughes, *No Time for Tears*, pp. 261–62; see also Belinda Jelliffe, *For Dear Life* (New York: Charles Scribner's Sons, 1936), p. 286.

16. Parsons, *Nursing Problems*, pp. 5–6; Aikens, *Studies in Ethics*, p. 280.

17. Brunettie Burrow, *Angels in White* (San Antonio, Tex.: Naylor, 1959), pp. 11–19, 23; Ida May Hadden, *First and Second Chronicles* (New York: Fleming H. Revell, 1937), p. 73; Lara Hartwell, "The Returned Nurse," *AJN* 20 (Jan. 1920): 294–96; quoted in Burgess, *Nurses, Patients*, p. 326.

18. Josephine Goldmark, *Nursing and Nursing Education in the United States: A Report of the Committee for the Study of Nursing Education* (New York: Macmillan, 1923), p. 168.

19. Burgess, *Nurses, Patients*, pp. 291–92.

20. See, for example, notices from Detroit, *AJN* 27 (Jan. 1927): 62; N.C., Fla., Ala., Calif., *AJN* 27 (March 1927): 195–96, 216; Orlando, Fla., *AJN* 29 (Jan. 1929): 91; Asheville, N.C., *AJN* 29 (June 1929): 730; Washington, D.C., *AJN* 28 (July 1928): 733.

21. May Ayres Burgess, "More Census Figures—the Whole United States," *AJN* 32 (May 1932): 516.

22. Burgess, *Nurses, Patients*, pp. 84–85, 131; letter from St. Petersburg, Fla., *AJN* 28 (Nov. 1928): 1148; "Too Many Nurses—Where?" *AJN* 29 (March 1929): 291–300.

23. Burgess, *Nurses, Patients*, pp. 296, 300, 301, 304, 307.

24. Ibid.,pp. 293–94; editorial, "Drudges," *AJN* 24 (March 1924): 462.

25. "The Life Story of One Private Duty Nurse," *AJN* 27 (March 1927): 171–72.

26. Comparative data are from Winifred D. Wandersee, *Women's Work and Family Values, 1920–1940* (Cambridge, Mass.: Harvard Univ. Press, 1981), p. 11.

27. Quoted in Burgess, *Nurses, Patients*, p. 339.

28. Iva Marie Lowry, *Second Landing* (Philadelphia: Dorrance, 1974).

29. Harriet A. Byrne, "The Age Factor as It Relates to Women in Business and the Professions," U.S. Dept. of Labor, Women's Bureau (Washington, D.C.: G.P.O., 1934), p. 2; Wandersee, *Women's Work and Family Values*, pp. 35–38; C.-E.A. Winslow, "Nursing and the Community," *Public Health Nursing* 30 (April 1938): 234–35.

30. Burgess, *Nurses, Patients*, p. 191; Minnie S. Hollingsworth, "The Work of the Private Duty Nurse Today," *AJN* 21 (July 1921): 704; Frances Ott, "Where Are We Going in Private Duty?" *TNHR* 83 (July 1929): 200–204; "Calls for Non-Professional Workers Increase," *AJN* 44 (May 1944): 478.

31. Burgess, *Nurses, Patients*, p. 145. Susan Reverby's study of a Boston registry in the 1880s and 1890s also documents the graduate nurse's advantage. See " 'Neither for the Drawing Room nor for the Kitchen . . . ': Private Duty Nurses, 1873–1914," paper presented at the Organization of American Historians convention, April 1978.

32. Many commented on the demoralizing effects of this lack of standards and the absence of a career ladder in private duty; see, for example, Goldmark, *Nursing and Nursing Education*, pp. 169–70; "Changing Frontiers in Private Duty Nursing," *TNHR* 106 (March 1941): 189–91.

33. Grace M. Cook, "Central Directories and Their Relation to Private Duty Nursing," *AJN* 21 (Dec. 1920): 148–51; "The Value of a Local Directory," *AJN* 22 (Sept. 1922): 1021; Burgess, *Nurses, Patients*, p. 515; Janet M. Geister, "Should Nurses Plan or Drift?" *TNHR* 94 (Feb. 1935): 129–32; "Centralized Official Registries for Nurses," *TNHR* 79 (Aug. 1927): 144–46; Geister, "Private Duty Nurses, Will You Do It?" *TNHR* 94 (March 1935): 219–21. Quotation from Jessie J. Turnbull, "The Paucity of Nurses as One of the Challenges of a Hospital," American Hospital Association *Proceedings* (1926), p. 60.

34. For a more detailed discussion of the registry plan and an analysis of Janet M. Geister, a loyal supporter of private-duty nurses, see Susan Reverby, " 'Something Besides Waiting': The Politics of Private Duty Nursing Reform in the Depression," in Ellen Condliffe Lagemann, ed., *Nursing*

History: New Perspectives, New Possibilities (New York: Teachers College Press, forthcoming).

35. Letter from Mary T., R.N., Michigan, *TNHR* 72 (April 1924): 386.

36. "Registries and Placement Bureaus," *TNHR* 97 (Aug. 1936): 146.

37. Claribel A. Wheeler, "The Function of the Private Duty Nurse in the Community," *AJN* 25 (March 1925): 201; Augusta M. Condit, "Who Makes the Best Hourly Nurse?" *AJN* 30 (Jan. 1930): 31–32; Shirley C. Titus, "Group Nursing," *AJN* 30 (July 1930): 845–50; "Highlights of the Biennial," *AJN* 30 (July 1930): 916–17; Rhoda Wickwire, "Forecast for Private Duty Nursing," *AJN* 37 (March 1937): 245.

38. Quoted in Burgess, *Nurses, Patients*, p. 351; and see other examples, pp. 351–52.

39. See, for example, Adda Eldridge, "Objectives for Private Duty Sections," *AJN* 23 (April 1923): 539–40; Alma Ham Scott, "Private Duty Sections," *AJN* 33 (June 1933): 549–55; Geister, "Private Duty Nurses, Will You Do It?"

40. Gertrude B. Redmond, "The Challenge of a Private Duty Nurse," *AJN* 37 (Jan. 1937): 6–7; Mary F. Wallace, "Some Problems of Private Duty Nursing," *AJN* 30 (April 1930): 451–55; Laura Davidson Wall, "About Face," *AJN* 37 (Sept. 1937): 986.

41. Ott, "Where Are We Going?" p. 204.

42. Marion H. Addington, "Cooperation between the Private Duty Nurse and the Hospital," *AJN* 31 (Jan. 1931): 40, 43; Burgess, *Nurses, Patients*, pp. 416, 391–93; Zula Pasley, "Something Can Be Done," *TNHR* 79 (Dec. 1927): 617.

43. "Nurses Emancipated," *TNHR* 102 (Feb. 1939): 123; letter from C. B., Detroit, *TNHR* 115 (July 1945): 6; letter from Grace Wilkins, San Francisco, *RN* 3 (Jan. 1940): 2.

44. Letter from Ohio nurse, *TNHR* 114 (Jan. 1945): 40.

45. "High Lights of the Biennial," *AJN* 30 (July 1930): 921–27; Alma H. Scott, "Questions," *AJN* 31 (March 1931): 336; Geister, "Is the Private Duty Nurse Standing Still?" *TNHR* 98 (Jan. 1937): 31–35, 52; letter from J. M. G. [Geister?], "Are We Embalmed?" *TNHR* 98 (March 1937): 290.

46. Letter from E. K., Mass., *AJN* 20 (Jan. 1920): 331; "What Does She Want?" *TNHR* 85 (Dec. 1930): 775 (emphasis in original).

47. Letter From H. A. H., *TNHR* 67 (July 1921): 48–49; *TNHR* 68 (Feb. 1922): 123; A Laywoman, "Nurses as I Have Known Them," *AJN* 20 (July 1920): 794.

48. Editorial, "The Voice of Experience," *AJN* 36 (Feb. 1936): 159; Jane M. Holbrow, "Some Problems in Nursing an Aged Patient," *AJN* 31 (Feb. 1931): 174–75; obituary, "Clara H. Treglown," *AJN* 39 (March 1939): 333.

49. "Nursing as a Business," *TNHR* 65 (Nov. 1920): 419–20.

50. Letter from "Ex-U.S.N. Nurse," *AJN* 21 (Dec. 1920): 182–83; quotations from Burgess, *Nurses, Patients,* pp. 327, 329, 350, 332.

51. Burgess, *Nurses, Patients,* pp. 311–13, 334; Jelliffe, *For Dear Life,* p. 353.

52. Hughes, *No Time for Tears;* similar accounts appear in Jelliffe, *For Dear Life,* and Corinne Johnson Kern, *I Go Nursing* (New York: E. P. Dutton, 1933).

53. Burgess, *Nurses, Patients,* p. 148; Margaret C. Klem, "Who Purchase Private Duty Nursing Services?" *AJN* 39 (Oct. 1939): 1069–77; see also editorial, *AJN* 35 (Jan. 1935): 56.

54. Dorothy Parker, "Horsie," in *After Such Pleasures* (New York: Viking, 1933), pp. 3–4.

55. Ibid., p. 6.

56. Burgess, *Nurses, Patients,* pp. 76, 98; "The Registry Looks at the Private Duty Nurse," *AJN* 29 (Dec. 1929): 1465; "Our Mutual Obligation to Nursing," *AJN* 38 (Feb. 1938): 193; and see also Habel and Milton, *The Graduate Nurse in the Home,* p. vii. This manual was written in 1939, in response to the "problem" of the private-duty nurse in the home. The authors noted case-selecting with disapproval, and indicated that nurses were somewhat less able to avoid home cases in the depression years.

57. Burgess, *Nurses, Patients,* p. 353.

58. Letter from Zula Shorey, "Private Duty Nurses, We Challenge You!" *AJN* 42 (Aug. 1942): 945–46; editorial, "Private Duty Nursing in War-Time," *AJN* 42 (Oct. 1942): 1171; editorial, "Have You Thought It Through, Private Duty Nurses?" *AJN* 43 (June 1943): 522; Edwiga S. Rafalowska, "Private Duty Nursing in Wartime," *AJN* 43 (Sept. 1943): 820; "Miss Merling Saves One for Uncle Sam," *AJN* 43 (Nov. 1943): 1020–21. *AJN* announced the War Manpower Commission's classification of private-duty nurses as non-essential in "Criteria of Essentiality for Nurses," *AJN* 43 (Nov. 1943): 977–79. For move to hospital jobs, see Pearl McIver, "Registered Nurses in the United States," *AJN* 42 (July 1942): 769–73.

59. Eli Ginzberg, *A Program for the Nursing Profession* (New York: Macmillan, 1948), p. 33; Everett C. Hughes, Helen MacGill Hughes, and Irwin Deutscher, *Twenty Thousand Nurses Tell Their Story* (Philadelphia: Lippincott, 1958), p. 253; interview with Ruth I., 25 Oct. 1976.

CHAPTER 4

1. Isabel W. Lowman, editorial, *Public Health Nursing* (hereafter cited as *PHN*) 15 (Feb. 1923): 55; Sally Lucas Jean, "The Nurse and the School Child," *PHN* 15 (Jan. 1923): 9; and see also Michael M. Davis, Jr., *Immigrant Health and the Community* (New York: Harper and Brothers, 1921), p. 3.

2. Annie M. Brainard, *The Evolution of Public Health Nursing* (Philadelphia: W. B. Saunders, 1922), pp. 215–16, 253–57.

3. For histories of public health, see C.-E.A. Winslow, *The Evolution and Significance of the Modern Public Health Campaign* (New Haven, Conn.: Yale Univ. Press, 1923); George Rosen, *A History of Public Health* (New York: MD Publications, 1958); Rosen, *From Medical Police to Social Medicine* (New York: Science History Publications, 1974); Rosen, *Preventive Medicine in the United States, 1900–1975: Trends and Interpretations* (New York: Prodist, 1977); Barbara Guttman Rosenkrantz, *Public Health and the State: Changing Views in Massachusetts, 1842–1936* (Cambridge, Mass.: Harvard Univ. Press, 1972); James H. Cassedy, *Charles V. Chapin and the Public Health Movement* (Cambridge, Mass.: Harvard Univ. Press, 1962).

4. Brainard, *Evolution*, pp. 280–81; Richard Harrison Shryock, *National Tuberculosis Association, 1904–1954* (New York: Arno, 1977; first published in 1957); Samuel Haber, *Efficiency and Uplift: Scientific Management in the Progressive Era, 1890–1920* (Chicago: Univ. of Chicago Press, 1964); J. Stanley Lemons, *The Woman Citizen: Social Feminism in the 1920s* (Urbana, Ill.: Univ. of Illinois Press, 1973).

5. Brainard, *Evolution*, pp. 240, 304.

6. Emma Moynihan, "Public Health and Child Welfare," *PHN* 12 (Jan. 1920): 56.

7. Brainard, *Evolution*, pp. 300–303.

8. Mary Sewall Gardner, *Public Health Nursing*, 2nd ed. (New York: Macmillan, 1933; 1st ed., 1916), p. 387. See also Thomas Parran, *Shadow on the Land* (New York: Reynal and Hitchcock, 1937).

9. Surveys conducted in 1924 and 1934 by the National Organization for Public Health Nursing (NOPHN) indicated that maternity and infant-care programs were the most common and best organized of all public-health nursing services. See NOPHN, *Committee to Study Visiting Nursing* (New York, 1924), pp. 24, 26; and NOPHN, *Survey of Public Health Nursing: Administration and Practice* (New York: The Commonwealth Fund, 1934), pp. 29–30, 34–35, 162. For more information on Sheppard-Towner, see Lemons, *The Woman Citizen*.

10. "Who Pays for Public Health Nursing?" *PHN* 18 (May 1926): 261; Amelia Howe Grant, *Nursing: A Community Health Service* (Philadelphia: W. B. Saunders, 1942), p. 18; Louise M. Tattershall, "Census of Public Health Nursing in the United States—1924," *PHN* 18 (Jan. 1926): 24–27; May Ayres Burgess, *Nurses, Patients, and Pocketbooks: Report of a Study of the Economics of Nursing* (New York: Committee on the Grading of Nursing Schools, 1928), p. 249.

11. For a detailed history and interpretation of the NOPHN, see M. Louise Fitzpatrick, *The National Organization for Public Health Nursing, 1912–1952: Development of a Practice Field* (New York: National League for Nursing, 1975).

12. Brainard, *Evolution*, p. 340; Gardner, *Public Health Nursing*, p. 257.

13. Gardner, *Public Health Nursing*, p. 255; Mary Beard, *The Nurse in Public Health* (New York: Harper and Brothers, 1929), pp. 88, 89; Evelina Reed, "The Public Health Nurse and the Job," *PHN* 12 (Dec. 1920): 1016.

14. Fitzpatrick, *NOPHN*, pp. 90–91, 96, 126, 174–75.

15. NOPHN, *Survey* (1934), p. 17; for a later comparison, see Hortense Hilbert, "Public Health Nursing Services in Clinics," *PHN* 36 (May 1944): 209–10.

16. Burgess, *Nurses, Patients*, pp. 252, 254.

17. Quoted in Burgess, *Nurses, Patients*, pp. 117–18; Davis, *Immigrant Health*, pp. 285–88; for information on black nurses in public health, see Fitzpatrick, *NOPHN*, pp. 88–89.

18. Gardner, *Public Health Nursing*, p. 48; Sara E. Parsons, *Nursing Problems and Obligations* (Boston: Whitcomb and Barrows, 1916), p. 147; *Maternity Handbook for Pregnant Mothers and Expectant Fathers* (New York: Maternity Center Association, 1932), pp. 28–45; "Two 'Health Essays,' " *PHN* 15 (Oct. 1923): 504; Red Cross campaign posters, Smithsonian Institution.

19. Mary Breckinridge, *Wide Neighborhoods: A Story of the Frontier Nursing Service* (New York: Harper and Brothers, 1952), p. 242; Gardner, *Public Health Nursing*, p. 43. See also Beard, *The Nurse in Public Health*, p. 3.

20. Manuals and articles in *PHN* outlined the procedures for obtaining standing orders and emphasized their importance. See Florence Swift Wright, *Industrial Nursing: For Industrial, Public Health and Pupil Nurses, and for Employers of Labor* (New York: Macmillan, 1919), p. 26; "Standing Orders for Health Education," *PHN* 22 (March 1930): 138; Violet H. Hodgson, *Public Health Nursing in Industry* (New York: Macmillan, 1933), p. 32; NOPHN, *Manual of Public Health Nursing* (New York: Macmillan, 1939), pp. 10–13, 140; Grant, *Nursing: A Community Health Service*, p. 53; Bethel J. McGrath, *Nursing in Commerce and Industry* (New York: The Commonwealth Fund, 1946), p. 51. Information on informality of doctors' supervision in bedside nursing from interview with Jane G., 29 Dec. 1976.

21. E. C. Miller, "Nursing in a Camp for Homeless Men," *PHN* 26 (Nov. 1934): 594; Elinor D. Gregg, *The Indians and the Nurse* (Norman, Okla.: Univ. of Oklahoma Press, 1965), p. 162.

22. NOPHN, *Visiting Nursing*, p. 22; NOPHN, *Survey*, pp. 127, 130; "Medical Relationships in Non-Official PHNAs," *PHN* 26 (Nov. 1934): 574.

23. Gardner, *Public Health Nursing*, p. 184; Florence Swift Wright, "Constructive Supervision of Midwives," *PHN* 12 (Feb. 1920): 124; Marguerite Bonar, "The Tuberculosis Nurse in a Public Health Program," *PHN* 15 (Feb. 1923): 86; Helen W. Kelly, "Some Observations on Rural Work," *PHN* 13 (Jan. 1921): 18.

24. Borden S. Veeder, M.D., "Problems in Connection with the

Administration of Well-Baby Clinics," *PHN* 17 (Feb. 1925): 61; "Inter-dependence of Physicians and Public Health Nurses in Community Health Work," *PHN* 16 (Sept. 1924): 452; Gregg, *The Indians and the Nurse*, p. 27.

25. Mary V. Paguad, "Problems in Connection with the Administration of Well-Baby Clinics,"*PHN* 17 (Jan. 1925): 17–19.

26. Merrill Champion, M.D., "Again, What of the Public Health Nurse?" *PHN* 15 (Feb. 1923): 69; Isabel W. Lowman, editorial, *PHN* 15 (Feb. 1923): 55–56.

27. NOPHN, *Survey* (1934), p. 131; the same source also notes "the rather universal objection to free clinics or conferences sponsored by any agency"(pp. 24–25). See also John Duffy, "The American Medical Profession and Public Health: From Support to Ambivalence," *Bulletin of the History of Medicine* 53 (spring 1979): 1–22.

28. Moynihan, "Public Health and Child Welfare," p. 59.

29. Gardner, *Public Health Nursing*, p. 184; "Medical Relationships in Non-Official PHNAs," *PHN* 26 (Nov. 1934): 574; Annie M. Brainard, *Organization of Public Health Nursing* (New York: Macmillan, 1919), pp. 71–72; Beard, *The Nurse in Public Health*, p. 76; NOPHN, *Survey* (1934), p. 15.

30. Dorothy Bird Nyswander, *Solving School Health Problems* (New York: The Commonwealth Fund, 1942), pp. 88–89; Gardner, *Public Health Nursing*, p. 153; Beard, *The Nurse in Public Health*, p. 48.

31. Davis, *Immigrant Health*, p. 3.

32. Ivan Illich, *Medical Nemesis: The Expropriation of Health* (New York: Pantheon, 1976).

33. Mabelle S. Welsh, "Campaigning against Pediculosis," *PHN* 16 (Aug. 1924): 387; "Making Billy Safe for Democracy" and "Making Better Americans," *PHN* 21 (Jan. 1929): 36–40; Marie L. Rose, "Some Examples of Vitalized Health Teaching," *PHN* 13 (Sept. 1921): 449.

34. Edith E. Young, "A Day in the Baby Clinic," *PHN* 13 (July 1921): 333; Marguerite Wales, *The Public Health Nurse in Action* (New York: Macmillan, 1941), pp. 425–27; *Maternity Handbook*, pp. 82, 85, 93, 103, 157–58, 174–76; "Standards of Habit Formation," *PHN* 22 (Feb. 1930): 77.

35. Cora Baertsch, "School Nursing on a State-wide Plan," *PHN* 17 (Feb. 1925): 89.

36. See, for example, Bertha M. Wood, "Foods of the Foreign Born," *PHN* 22 (April 1930): 207–8; interview with Jane G., 29 Dec. 1976.

37. "Infant Feeding Trials in the Mountains," *PHN* 19 (July 1927): 368–69. Articles on working with midwives appeared frequently in the 1920s and 1930s; for examples, see Wright, "Constructive Supervision of Midwives," pp. 121–26; "A County Midwife Class," *PHN* 18 (Jan. 1926): 22–23; Lalla Mary Goggans, "Florida's First Institute for Midwives," *PHN* 26 (March 1934): 133–36. Ruth Gilbert, *The Public Health Nurse and Her Patient* (New York: The Commonwealth Fund, 1940), p. 162.

38. Gregg, *The Indians and the Nurse*, p. 3; "Health Examination for Everyone!" *PHN* 15 (Sept. 1923): 452–54; Anne Stevens, "The Public Health Nurse and the Extension of Maternity Nursing," *PHN* 12 (June 1920): 498; Mary Bliss Dickinson, "Little Mothers' Leagues," *PHN* 12 (July 1920): 602–3; Mary Scudder McDermott, "A Summer Time Suggestion," *PHN* 15 (Aug. 1923): 423–24; Louise Franklin Bache, *Health Education in an American City* (Garden City, N.Y.: Doubleday, Doran, 1934).

39. Paul Stevens, "Tonsils and Tact," *Hygeia* 13, no. 3 (March 1935): 356–58; Wales, *Public Health Nurse in Action*, p. 93; Pattie R. Saunders, "Neblett's Landing," *PHN* 29 (June 1937): 387–88.

40. Brainard, *Organization of Public Health Nursing*, p. 31; Beard, *The Nurse in Public Health*, pp. 52–59; Lillian D. Wald, *Windows on Henry Street* (Boston: Little, Brown, 1934), pp. 91–92.

41. Quoted in Harriet B. Cook, "Undergraduate Affiliation in Public Health Nursing in a County," *PHN* 27 (Feb. 1935): 72; "Here Comes the Nurse!" *PHN* 41 (Aug. 1949): 448–50; Lillian D. Wald, *The House on Henry Street* (New York: Henry Holt, 1915), and Wald, *Windows on Henry Street*; interview with Jane G., 29 Dec. 1976.

42. Harriet Leck, "Charge to a Graduating Class," *PHN* 12 (Aug. 1920): 686; Edna L. Foley, "A Definition of Nursing," *PHN* 13 (Feb. 1921): 62.

43. Glee L. Hastings, "Some Emotional Problems of Public Health Nurses," *PHN* 24 (Dec. 1932): 659–60; Burgess, *Nurses, Patients*, pp. 257, 269–70.

44. Reed, "The Public Health Nurse," p. 1017; Gardner, *Public Health Nursing*, p. 181; NOPHN, *Manual*, p. 35.

45. See note 9 above.

46. Brainard, *Evolution*, p. 420.

47. Committee on the Costs of Medical Care, *Medical Care for the American People* (Chicago: Univ. of Chicago Press, 1932), p. 42; Julius B. Richmond, *Currents in American Medicine* (Cambridge, Mass.: Harvard Univ. Press, 1969), pp. 11–20; Lloyd C. Taylor, Jr., *The Medical Profession and Social Reform, 1885–1945* (New York: St. Martin's Press, 1974), pp. 121–27.

48. "What Happened to Public Health Nursing in 1933," *PHN* 26 (Sept. 1934), 452; "Vocational Placement," *PHN* 25 (March 1933): 149; Louise M. Tattershall, "Changes in the Public Health Nursing Field during 1932," *PHN* 25 (April 1933): 216; Katherine Tucker, "Activities of the NOPHN," *PHN* 23 (Jan. 1931): 29; "Can You Stand Alone?" *PHN* 23 (Oct. 1931): 461; "Meet the Crisis!" *PHN* 24 (Dec. 1932): 651–52; Alma C. Haupt, "Some New Emphases in Public Health Nursing," *PHN* 27 (Dec. 1935): 626.

49. Marion W. Sheahan, "An Experiment in Double Relief," *PHN* 25 (July 1933): 380; Ellen S. Woodward, "Federal Aspects of Unemployment

among Professional Women," *PHN* 26 (June 1934): 300; "WPA Nursing Projects," *PHN* 29 (Jan. 1937): 50; Nina Barton, "Experiences of an ERA Nurse," *PHN* 26 (Dec. 1934): 665–67; Laura A. Draper, "Effect of ERA on 921)Local Programs," *PHN* 28 (May 1936): 310; Matilda Ann Wade, "Community Nursing—FSA Style," *PHN* 34 (Feb. 1942): 82–88.

50. "The Significance of the FERA Programs to Public Health Nursing," *PHN* 26 (Oct. 1934): 517; "Not Just Any Nurse, Please!" *PHN* 29 (March 1937): 139–40; "Civil Works Projects," *PHN* 26 (April 1934): 175–77; "SERA Activities in Public Health Nursing," *PHN* 27 (May 1935): 266; Haupt, "Some New Emphases," p. 628.

51. "Public Health Nursing under the Social Security Act," *PHN* 28 (Sept. 1936): 583; Anna L. Tittman, "New Jobs for Old," *PHN* 30 (Jan, 1938): 11; "Better Care for Mothers and Babies," *PHN* 30 (Feb. 1938): 71–73; Mabel Reid, "1938 Census of Public Health Nurses," *PHN* 30 (Nov. 1938): 632–35; "Official Agency Support," *PHN* 40 (Feb. 1948): 60.

52. Anne R. Winslow, "The Private Agency in Today's Health Program," *PHN* 29 (Apr. 1937): 204–7; Linn Brandenberg, "Financing Voluntary Public Health Nursing Agencies," *PHN* 40 (Aug. 1948): 394.

53. "Hospital Mothers' Classes," *PHN* 25 (Jan. 1933): 38; Constance Roy, "A VNA Assists with Integration," *PHN* 37 (July 1945): 353–55; "Our Annual Inventory," *PHN* 27 (Oct. 1935): 523; Katherine Faville, "Private Agency in the Defense Program," *PHN* 33 (Jan. 1942): 4–10.

54. "Rural Hospitals as Health Centers," *PHN* 22 (Feb. 1930): 86–87; "Interrelationship of Visiting Nurse Service and Hospital," *PHN* 22 (Feb. 1930): 88–91; "Public Health Nursing under the Englewood Plan," *PHN* 22 (Mar. 1930): 126–34; "Experiment in Hospital Social Service Work by Public Health Nurses," *PHN* 24 (Nov. 1932): 626–28; Basil C. McLean, "The Hospital as a Community Health Agency," *PHN* 40 (March 1948): 115–18; Graham L. Davis, "The Hospital as a Community Health Center," *PHN* 40 (June 1948): 311–14; Joseph W. Mountin, "The Future of Public Health Nursing," *PHN* 37 (Nov. 1945): 542–47.

55. "Public Health Nursing Service in Clinics," *PHN* 36 (May 1944): 210; John H. Stokes, "Public Health and Social Hygiene," *PHN* 26 (Oct. 1934): 535; Charlotte M. Inglesby, "A Teaching Clinic for Syphilis and Gonorrhea," *PHN* 28 (Feb. 1936): 104; Karen E. Munch, "Nurse Interview in the Tuberculosis Clinic," *PHN* 38 (Feb. 1946): 73–76.

56. Agnes Fuller, "More about Wartime Adjustments," *PHN* 37 (May 1945): 242–45; Dorothy E. Wiesner and Margaret M. Murphy, "Inactive Nurses and Auxiliary Workers," *PHN* 36 (March 1944): 142–43; Hortense Hilbert, "Public Health Nursing Services in Clinics," *PHN* 36 (May 1944): 211; Alberta B. Wilson, "Using Emergency Personnel," *PHN* 36 (March 1944): 137–41; Thomas W. Scott, "Application of Certain Business Methods to Nursing Organizations," *PHN* 35 (July 1943): 367–74; "The

School Nurse and Civilian Defense," *PHN* 34 (April 1942): 204; Grace Ross, "An Official Agency Saves Nursing Time," *PHN* 37 (May 1945): 249–51; The Nurse's Aid in the Visiting Nurses' Association," *PHN* 35 (Dec. 1943): 678, 684.

57. Ruth Farrisey, "Supervising the Practical Nurse," *PHN* 40 (June 1948): 321; Elizabeth C. Phillips, "Practical Nurses—Of Course We Employ Them!" *PHN* 42 (Dec. 1950): 663–67; see also Jessie M. Dawson, "The Public Health Assistant in a Health Department Program," *PHN* 44 (Aug. 1952): 443–44.

58. Marie L. Johnson, "Public Health Nursing Administration in the Changing Order," *PHN* 39 (July 1947): 333–36; Lois Blakey, "Relation of Psychiatric Social Work to Public Health Nursing," *PHN* 22 (Jan. 1930): 26–30; C.-E. A. Winslow, "The Voluntary Nursing Agency," *PHN* 38 (Nov. 1946): 609; Betty B. Bloom, "The Public Health Nurse and the Medical-Social Consultant," *Nursing Outlook* (hereafter cited as *N. Outlook*) 1 (March 1953): 150–51; Eleanor W. Mole, "The Patient Goes Home from the Hospital—So What!" *PHN* 39 (Jan. 1947): 30–34.

59. Alice Warinner, "Psychiatric Social Worker as Consultant," *PHN* 41 (July 1949): 395; letter from R.N., New York, *N. Outlook* 2 (July 1954): 344; letter from Margaret L. Shetland, Syracuse, N.Y., *N. Outlook* 2 (Oct. 1954): 560.

60. Mary A. Barke, "Extra-Familial Contact Tracing," *PHN* 35 (Jan. 1943): 16; "Where Has It Been Done?" *PHN* 34 (Nov. 1942): 601; Ruth W. Hubbard, "Role of the Voluntary Nursing Agency," *PHN* 40 (Jan. 1948): 6; Review of Theda L. Waterman, *Nursing For Community Health*, *PHN* 39 (Dec. 1947): 627.

61. Nursing Information Bureau, *Facts about Nursing* (New York: American Nurses' Association, 1950), pp. 13, 21–22; Mary Ella Chayer, "Shall We Teach Them All to Fly?" *PHN* 41 (July 1949): 369–72. For the NOPHN's consistent policy of postgraduate credentials, see Fitzpatrick, *NOPHN*, pp. 48–49, 79–81, 86, 129.

62. Sybil H. Pease, "The Interview in Public Health Nursing," *PHN* 25 (March 1933): 137; Elizabeth I. Adamson, "Function of the Public Health Nurse," *PHN* 26 (Oct. 1934): 545; Lucile Petry, "Community Needs for Nursing Care," *PHN* 40 (Aug. 1948): 392.

63. Roscoe P. Kandle, "Changing Aspects of Public Health," *N. Outlook* 1 (July 1953): 384–86; Elisabeth Cogswell Phillips, "Chronic Illness and the Nurse," *PHN* 39 (Feb. 1947): 87–91; Frederic D. Zeman, "The Medical Significance of Our Aging Population," *PHN* 41 (July 1949): 381–84; Hortense Hilbert, "Extending Hospital Care to the Home," *PHN* 41 (July 1949): 378–80; Martha D. Adams, "A Nursing Director's Dilemma," *N. Outlook* 2 (Nov. 1954): 575–77.

64. Donald B. Armstrong, "A 40 Year Demonstration of Public

Health Nursing by the Metropolitan Life Insurance," *PHN* 43 (Jan. 1951: 41–44; Alma Gaines Ramsey, "The End of an Era," *PHN* 44 (June 1952): 318–20, 324.

65. Irma E. Reeve, "Nursing the Chronically Ill," *PHN* 39 (Dec. 1947): 618.

66. Ruth Fisher and Alma C. Haupt, "Community Efforts to Provide Visiting Nurse Service, *N. Outlook* 1 (Jan. 1953): 46–48; Martha Adams, "Adjustments in Visiting Nursing Associations," *PHN* 44 (June 1952): 321–24; Franz Goldmann, "Nursing in Health Insurance Plans," *PHN* 40 (Aug. 1948): 405–8; Margaret C. Klem, "Nursing Opportunities in Medical Care Insurance," *PHN* 43 (Jan. 1951): 8–16; "A Report of a Study of the Effects of the Termination of Metropolitan Nursing Contracts," *PHN* 43 (May 1951): 285; Alice F. De Benneville, "Financing Voluntary Public Health Nursing Services," *N. Outlook* 2 (April 1954): 86.

67. Elizabeth G. Fox, "I Vote No," *PHN* 40 (Aug. 1948): 416–27; "Report," *PHN* 40 (Nov. 1948): 534; "Non-Nurse Agencies in the NLA," *PHN* 44 (Feb. 1952): 71–75; editorial, *PHN* 44 (June 1952): 307–8. In discussing the decline of the NOPHN, and elsewhere in her history, Fitzpatrick suggests that the organization may have been hampered by internal conflicts between leaders and other nurses. The NOPHN enrolled only about half of all public-health nurses, perhaps because of conflict over leaders' educational standards (see Fitzpatrick, *NOPHN*, pp. 90–91, 96, 126, 174–75, 205). This suggestion seems consistent with the general pattern of nurses' resistance to professionalization, although there is less evidence of conflict among public-health nurses than in the nursing field in general. I suspect that two aspects of public-health nursing account for this. First, the NOPHN was primarily a national organization, with the one voice of *Public Health Nursing*; non-public-health nurses had several journals and various local organizations in which to voice their opinions. *PHN* did not even have a letters column until the late 1930s. Second, because public-health nursing was an expanding field with many opportunities, dissenting nurses may not have felt threatened by the NOPHN's struggle for restrictive credentials.

68. René Dubos, *Mirage of Health: Utopias, Progress, and Biological Change* (Garden City, N.Y.: Doubleday, 1958), pp. 28–32; Illich, *Medical Nemesis*, pp. 15–22; Barbara Ehrenreich and Deirdre English, *For Her Own Good: 150 Years of the Experts' Advice to Women* (Garden City, N.Y.: Anchor/Doubleday, 1978), pp. 127–64, 190–239.

69. The slogan "every nurse a public health nurse" was quoted (and refuted) in Chayer, "Shall We Teach Them All to Fly?"

CHAPTER 5

1. "More General Staff Nurses," *American Journal of Nursing* (hereafter cited as *AJN*) 38 (Feb. 1938): 186–90; "Did You Ever See a Nurse *Nursing*?"

AJN 38 (April 1938): 30 (S); Beulah Amidon, *Better Nursing for America* (Public Affairs Pamphlets no. 60; New York: Public Affairs Committee, 1941), pp. 13–14; Everett C. Hughes, Helen MacGill Hughes, and Irwin Deutscher, *Twenty Thousand Nurses Tell Their Story* (Philadelphia: Lippincott, 1958), p. 258.

2. David Rosner, "Business at the Bedside: Health Care in Brooklyn, 1890–1915," in Susan Reverby and David Rosner, eds., *Health Care in America* (Philadelphia: Temple Univ. Press, 1979), pp. 117–31; Morris Vogel, *The Invention of the Modern Hospital: Boston, 1870–1930* (Chicago: Univ. of Chicago Press, 1980); Susan Reverby, "The Search for the Hospital Yardstick: Nursing and the Rationalization of Hospital Work," in Reverby and Rosner, *Health Care in America*, pp. 206–19.

3. A. E. Foote, "Simplification and Standardization," American Hospital Association *Proceedings* (1926), pp. 228–39.

4. David Rosner, "Social Control and Social Service: The Changing Use of Space in Charity Hospitals," *Radical History Review* 21 (fall 1979): 183–97.

5. John D. Thompson and Grace Goldin, *The Hospital: A Social and Architectural History (New Haven: Yale Univ. Press, 1975)*, especially ch. 7; "A Central Nourishment Kitchen," *AJN* 27 (Jan. 1927): 9–10; Theresa G. Ryan, "Central Trayroom Control," *AJN* 41 (March 1941): 313–14; Laura M. Grant, "A New Type of Nursing Unit," *AJN* 33 (March 1933): 2–7, 11; Martha Ruth Smith, "How to Evaluate Existing Nursing Procedures," *AJN* 30 (April 1930): 391–98; Thomas W. Scott, "Application of Certain Business Methods to Nursing Organizations," *Public Health Nursing* 35 (July 1943): 367–74.

6. W. D. Morse, M.D., "Standardization of Hospitals," *AJN* 27 (Feb. 1927): 111–14; "Report on the Committee on Training of Hospital Executives," American Hospital Association *Proceedings* (1925), pp. 410–11.

7. A. C. Bachmeyer, "Offer Course in Hospital Administration," *Hospital Management* 7 (Aug. 1919): 42–43.

8. A. C. Bachmeyer, "Qualifications and Training of Hospital Superintendents," *Modern Hospital* 18 (April 1922): 338–42; "Report," American Hospital Association *Proceedings* (1925), pp. 400–456; Arthur C. Bachmeyer and Gerhard Hartman, eds. *The Hospital in Modern Society* (New York: The Commonwealth Fund, 1943), pp. 115–32.

9. "Report," American Hospital Association *Proceedings* (1925), pp. 408, 400.

10. For cost studies comparing student and graduate staffs, see Robert E. Neff, "Cost of Nursing Service in the Hospital," *AJN* 30 (July 1930): 841–44; Phoebe Gordon, "Nursing Costs," *AJN* 30 (Nov. 1930): 1495–98; C. F. Neergaard, R. N. Brough, and A. M. MacNicol, "With or without a Training School: A Study of Nursing Costs," *AJN* 31 (Jan. 1931): 12–16; May Ayres Burgess, "What the Cost Study Showed," *AJN* 32 (April 1932): 427–32 (a summary of a survey of 218 schools); Rufus Rorem, "Is Student

Nursing a Real Economy?" *AJN* 33 (April 1933): 369–75. For studies comparing the efficiency of students and graduates, see National League of Nursing Education (NLNE), *A Study on the Use of Graduate Nurses for Bedside Nursing in the Hospital* (New York: NLNE, 1933), p. 54; Esther Thompson and Phoebe Gordon, "Student or Graduate Nurses' Service," *AJN* 31 (May 1931): 569–72.

11. "In 1932," *AJN* 33 (Jan. 1933): 3; E. H. L. Corwin, *The American Hospital* (New York: The Commonwealth Fund, 1946), p. 67; Ella A. Taylor, "Accredited Schools," *AJN* 35 (June 1935): 517–21.

12. In 1932 alone, hospitals added 239,157 beds and increased their capacities by 26 percent; see "In 1932," *AJN* 33 (Jan. 1933): 3; Philip A. Kalisch and Beatrice J. Kalisch, *The Advance of American Nursing* (Boston: Little, Brown, 1978), pp. 418–23, 438–41. For changing design of hospitals, see Thompson and Goldin, *The Hospital*, pp. 207, 213, 215–17.

13. May Ayres Burgess and William Darrach, *Nursing Schools—Today and Tomorrow: Final Report of the Committee on the Grading of Nursing Schools* (New York, 1934), p. 91; Katharine Appel Maroney, "How a Small Hospital Can Nurse Its Patients without a School," *AJN* 32 (June 1932): 640–42; Gertrude Strong Bates, "Graduate Nurses on a Staff Basis," *AJN* 33 (Aug. 1933): 755–56 (work-sharing at Ellis Hospital in Schenectady, N.Y.); Anna Kaplan, "Work-sharing at Beth Israel Hospital," *AJN* 33 (Jan. 1933): 36.

14. Pearl McIver, "Registered Nurses in the United States," *AJN* 42 (July 1942): 769–73; and see note 1 above.

15. Reverby, "Search for the Hospital Yardstick," argues that nurses themselves aggressively pursued rationalization; I have emphasized the divisions between leaders and others on the issue and have portrayed leaders as more ambivalent.

16. May Ayres Burgess, *Nurses, Patients, and Pocketbooks: Report of a Study of the Economics of Nursing* (New York: Committee on the Grading of Nursing Schools, 1928), pp. 390–91.

17. Celia Cranz, "Economic Aspects of General Duty," *AJN* 30 (Nov. 1930): 1499–1500; "Graduate vs. Student Staff," *AJN* 39 (Nov. 1939): 1258. See also Burgess, *Nurses, Patients*, pp. 410–12, 416.

18. Daniel Nelson, *Managers and Workers: Origins of the New Factory System in the United States, 1880–1920* (Madison: Univ. of Wisconsin Press, 1975).

19. "Official Registries and Professional Progress," *AJN* 26 (Feb. 1926): 93; Adda Eldredge, "Some Vocational Problems," *AJN* 37 (July 1937): 725; Carrie May Dokken, "The General Staff Nurse," *AJN* 38 (Feb. 1938): 143–46; Sister M. Bernice Beck, "General Staff Nursing," *AJN* 37 (Jan. 1937): 57–63; Elizabeth M. Jamieson, "The General Duty Nurse," *AJN* 29 (July 1929): 834–37; letter from a director of nursing, *Trained Nurse and Hospital Review* (hereafter cited as *TNHR*) 108 (Jan. 1942): 61.

20. "Graduate Staff Nursing," *AJN* 36 (June 1936): 591–96; letter, *AJN* 36 (Aug. 1936): 851; letter and editorial note, *AJN* 39 (April 1939): 435.

21. "Graduate Staff Nursing," *AJN* 36 (June 1936): 591–96; letter from "Private Duty," *TNHR* 100 (Feb. 1938): 167. See also "3,000 General Staff Nurses," *AJN* 41 (April 1941): 422–25; Sylvia M. Wetzel, "I Don't Like Nurses' Homes," *TNHR* 100 (Jan. 1938): 51–52; letter, *AJN* 41 (Oct. 1941): 1176; letter, *AJN* 42 (Nov. 1942): 1312; "Let's Consider the Staff Nurse, by One of Them," *AJN* 42 (May 1942): 52–53.

22. "Accidents to Nurses," *AJN* 41 (May 1941): 561–64; "Study Your Troubles!" *AJN* 29 (Sept. 1929): 1097–98. For other examples, see note 5 above.

23. Chelly Wassenberg and Ethel Northan, "Some Time Studies in Obstetrical Nursing," *AJN* 27 (July 1927): 544–55; Gladys Sellew, "A Time Study," *AJN* 29 (Jan. 1929): 79–83; National League of Nursing Education, *Manual of the Essentials of Good Hospital Nursing Service* (New York: NLNE, 1936), pp. 10–12.

24. "Graduates vs. Students," *AJN* 33 (May 1933): 479; Evelyn Nuyman Blier, "Orientation or Irritation?" *TNHR* 102 (March 1939): 240–43.

25. J. M. G[eister], "An Open Letter on Staff Nursing," *TNHR* 106 (April 1941): 362; letter, *AJN* 41 (Dec. 1941): 1448; letter from "Illinois nurse," *AJN* 27 (May 1927): 391; A. Faith Ankeny, "The Standpoint of a Nurse," *TNHR* 81 (Nov. 1928): 558. See also letter from R.N., Aberdeen, Wash., *RN* 1 (July 1938): 3–4.

26. "Graduates vs. Students," *AJN* 33 (May 1933): 479.

27. Annette Fiske, "Is Procedure Standardization Desirable?" *TNHR* 79 (Sept. 1927): 275–78; Fiske, "Will Standardization Promote Progress?" *TNHR* 80 (March 1928): 295–99. Quotations from letters are from "A Private Duty Nurse," *AJN* 30 (June 1930): 775 (emphasis in original) and letter, *AJN* 41 (Oct. 1941): 1176.

28. Burgess, *Nurses, Patients*, p. 468; Burgess and Darrach, *Nursing Schools*, pp. 101–2.

29. "Pressing Problems for Those in Private Duty," *TNHR* 97 (Aug. 1936): 141–42; this article discusses conflict over auxiliaries at the ANA convention and notes reluctance of NLNE to act on subsidiaries. NLNE, *Manual of the Essentials*, pp. 21–22; see also NLNE, *A Study of the Nursing Service in Fifty Selected Hospitals* (New York: United Hospital Fund, 1937), p. 360. Gradually, others began to emphasize that auxiliary workers should be licensed and regulated rather than removed from the workforce; see, for example, "The Registrar Said," *TNHR* 103 (July 1939): 72; Ella Hasenjaeger, "A Study of the Subsidiary Worker in New Jersey," *TNHR* 101 (Sept. 1938): 217–19.

30. Louise Kieninger, "The Subsidiary Worker," *AJN* 36 (Oct. 1936): 984–86; Mabel S. Campbell, "The Attendant's Place in One Hospital," *AJN*

39 (Feb. 1939): 161–64; Marion Wefer, "Susan Redmond, Army Nurse Corps Reserve," *TNHR* 121 (July 1948): 44–46.

3l. Susan Reverby, " 'Neither for the Drawing Room nor for the Kitchen . . . ': Private Duty Nurses, 1873–1914," paper presented at the Organization of American Historians convention, April 1978. Reverby's investigation of a Boston registry indicates that, despite their complaints, graduates enjoyed a distinct advantage over practicals in getting cases. See also Burgess, *Nurses, Patients*, pp. 145–47; doctors reported that they favored trained nurses over practicals. For an example of the perplexities of hospital division of labor, see Hilda M. Torrop, "How Much Nursing Service Should an Orderly Give?" *AJN* 37 (Jan. 1937): 15–17.

32. For examples of articles advocating rationalization to stretch out staffs, see M. Annie Leitch, "Using Heads to Save Feet," *TNHR* 107 (Sept. 1941): 184–85; editorial, "Staff Nurses to the Fore!" *AJN* 41 (Sept. 1941): 1055–67; Margaret E. Benson, "Meeting the Shortage of Nurses," *AJN* 41 (Dec. 1941): 1376–80.

33. "The Hospital Staff Nurse," *AJN* 41 (Jan. 1941): 55–56; "1943—a Stern and Terrible Year," *AJN* 43 (Jan. 1943): 2; "Recruiting Student Practical Nurses," *AJN* 44 (March 1944): 200–201; Dorothy Deming, "Practical Nurses—a Professional Responsibility," *AJN* 44 (Jan. 1944): 37.

34. "The Biennial," *AJN* 44 (July 1944): 629; Janet M. Geister, "Plain Talk," *TNHR* 113 (Dec. 1944): 441–43.

35. Quotations from letter from "Interested R.N.," *AJN* 48 (Sept. 1948): 6-adv.; letter from Marie Richard, R.N., La., *AJN* 47 (Jan. 1947): 48. See also Florence L. McQuillan, "We Need Standards of Nursing Care," *AJN* 47 (Feb. 1947): 77–79; letters from R.N., Calif., and M. K., R.N., Wash., *AJN* 46 (June 1946): 418; letter from "Nursing School Instructor," R.N., Calif., *AJN* 47 (Jan. 1947): 48.

36. Hilda M. Torrop, "More and Better," *RN* 10 (Jan. 1947): 54 (reports licensing laws for practical nurses in twenty states, with mandatory licensing in one); Nursing Information Bureau, *Facts about Nursing*, (New York: American Nurses' Association, 1955–56), p. 155 (reports licensure laws, most of them permissive, in effect throughout the U.S. except in Colo., W.Va., D.C.); Esther Lucile Brown, *Nursing for the Future* (New York: Russell Sage, 1948), p. 159.

37. Harry Braverman, *Labor and Monopoly Capital: The Degradation of Work in the Twentieth Century* (New York: Monthly Review Press, 1974). David Wagner argues that hospital work undercut nurses' skill and autonomy in "The Proletarianization of Nursing in the United States, 1932–1946," *International Journal of Health Services* 10 (1980): 271–90. In "The Search for the Hospital Yardstick," Susan Reverby suggests that nursing leaders saw rationalization as an opportunity.

38. "Tribute to an American War Nurse," *Army Nurse* 1 (July 1944): 5; Victor Robinson, *White Caps: The Story of Nursing* (Philadelphia: Lippin-

cott, 1946), p. 358. In an intriguing memoir, Army nurse Edith A. Aynes describes her battles with the war public relations bureau. She wanted the nurse presented as a professional; the bureau explicitly aimed to show the nurse as a woman and "morale booster." See *From Nightingale to Eagle* (Englewood Cliffs, N.J.: Prentice-Hall, 1973), p. 257.

39. The Red Cross voluntary aides ultimately became a source of wartime recruitment for paid auxiliaries, as discussed in "Red Cross Aides May Be Employed by Hospitals," *AJN* 44 (May 1944): 502; and Ida M. MacDonald, "Nurse's Aides for the Army," *AJN* 44 (July 1944): 659–60. For a statistical report of the widespread use of paid auxiliaries during the war, see Louise M. Tattershall and Marion E. Attenderfer, "Paid Auxiliary Nursing Workers Employed in General Hospitals," *AJN* 44 (Aug. 1944): 752–56.

40. For an excellent study of the rapid spread of this reorganization and of related medical innovations, see Louise B. Russell, "The Diffusion of New Hospital Technologies in the United States," *International Journal of Health Services* 6 (1976): 557–80.

41. For contemporary reports, see Rosemary Lucker, "Post-Anesthesia Recovery Room," *RN* 12 (June 1949): 44–45, 72, 74; "Post-Anesthesia Unit at Presbyterian Hospital," *TNHR* 121 (Oct. 1948): 196; "Special Care Unit for Seriously Ill Patients," *Nursing World* 130 (Dec. 1956): 6; J. Murray Beardsley, M.D., and Florence F. Carvisiglia, R.N., "A Special Care Ward for Surgical Patients," *Nursing World* 131 (March 1957): 11–13; Edward J. Thomas, "Progressive Patient Care," *Nursing World* 134 (March 1960): 11–12, 32; Hope Patterson, "How's Progressive Patient Care Doing?" *RN* 23 (April 1960): 62–68, 100–102. One article argued that intensive care units were a temporary expedient until private duty could be revived, as "it makes more sense to move nurses to sick people than sick people to nurses"; see "The ANA Convention Focuses on the Changing Role of Nurses," *Nursing World* 134 (July 1960): 13. Russell argues, as I do, that intensive care was initiated as a managerial strategy, and her data reveal the magnitude of administrators' miscalculations: in 1973, hospitals employed about 2.4 nurses for each ICU bed. See Russell, "Diffusion," pp. 570–72.

42. Temple Burling, Edith M. Lentz, and Robert N. Wilson, *The Give and Take in Hospitals* (New York: G. P. Putnam, 1956), p. 105.

43. See, for example, Doctor X, *Intern* (New York: Harper and Row, 1965); Elizabeth Morgan, *The Making of a Woman Surgeon* (New York: G. P. Putnam, 1980); the 1955 film *Not as a Stranger*, based on the Morton Thompson novel of the same name ("Make friends with the nurses," a senior doctor counsels his intern; "They run the hospital"). For a humorous and perceptive analysis of the informal negotiations that mediate this new relationship, see Leonard I. Stein, "The Doctor-Nurse Game," *Archives of General Psychiatry* 16 (June 1967): 699–703.

44. Interview with Astrid N., 23 Oct. 1976.

45. See, for example, Jon Franklin and Alan Doelp, *Shocktrauma* (New York: St. Martin's Press, 1980) and B. D. Colen, *Born at Risk* (New York: St. Martin's Press, 1981).

46. Quoted in Elizabeth Maury Dean, "One Hundred Who Were Private Duty Nurses," *AJN* 44 (June 1944): 560.

47. Ken Kesey, *One Flew over the Cuckoo's Nest* (New York: Penguin, 1976; first published in 1962).

48. T. K. Brown, "A Drink of Water," *O. Henry Awards Prize Stories, 1958* (Garden City, N.Y.: Doubleday, 1958), pp. 179–201; quotation is from p. 199.

49. For a more detailed interpretation of nurses in popular culture, see Barbara Melosh, "Doctors, Patients, and 'Big Nurse': Work and Gender in the Postwar Hospital," in Ellen Condliffe Lagemann, ed., *Nursing History: New Perspectives, New Possibilities* (New York: Teachers College Press, forthcoming).

50. Richard R. Lanese, *Authoritarianism in Nurses: Hospital-Significant Attitudes and Nursing Performance* (Columbus, Ohio: Systems Research Group, Engineering Experiment Station, 1961), pp. 42–43.

51. Editorial, "The Forgotten Woman," *RN* 1 (Dec. 1937): 22–23; "Ladies without Leisure," *RN* 1 (May 1938): 22; "For Better Staff Nursing," *RN* 2 (May 1939): 18–19.

52. Frances Elder, "Why Nurses Don't Stay Put," *RN* 21 (May 1958): 60–63; student poll reported in "Reviewing the News," *RN* 16 (Aug. 1953): 30–31. In *The Advance of American Nursing*, Kalisch and Kalisch implicitly accept the argument that nurses were responding to the domestic ideology of the 1950s. They argue that changing demography partly accounted for the nursing shortage (fewer young women than before), but also suggest that nurses withdrew from the workforce because of rising marriage and birth rates (see pp. 526–28).

53. Letter from Charles K. Ingram, Fort Lauderdale, Fla., *RN* 12 (Nov. 1948): 2–5; letter from R.N., N.Y., *RN* 12 (Aug. 1949): 5; Dorothy E. Travers, " . . . And Now I Am an Industrial Nurse," *RN* 14 (May 1951): 30–32, 68; "Is Collaboration Overdue?" *AJN* 47 (Feb. 1947): 65–67. See also letter from M. L. Paulding, Santa Maria, Calif., *RN* 9 (Jan. 1946): 18; Alice R. Clarke, "*RN* Speaks: Where Are We Going?" *RN* 10 (May 1947): 29; letter from Florence Brickett, East Orange, N.J., *RN* 13 (Feb. 1949): 10, 12.

54. On salary structures, see "Graduate Staff Nursing," *AJN* 36 (June 1936): 593; "Economic Status of the Nursing Profession," *AJN* 47 (July 1947): 460. Quotation from letter by Kate Janeke, Des Plaines, Ill., *RN* 19 (Feb. 1956): 10, 12. See also Martha Dudley, "Wanted: A Better Break for the Part-time Nurse," *RN* 22 (Aug. 1959): 33–36; letter from Jeanrose Williams, Kansas City, Ks., *RN* 16 (April 1954): 7; letter from Augustina B. Grady, N. Platte, Neb., *RN* 15 (April 1952): 8, 10; Roberta Michaels, "I

Take My Children to Work with Me!" *RN* 21 (July 1958): 44–47, 60–63; "No Baby Sitters Needed—One Hospital," *RN* 16 (April 1953): 58, 70.

55. Quotations from Janet M. Geister, "Candid Comments: Tomorrow Begins Today," *RN* 11 (Aug. 1948): 33–35, 76; Geister, "Displaced Nurses," *RN* 14 (April 1951): 33–36, 65. See also "*RN* Speaks: Nursing, the Stormy Petrel," *RN* 11 (Jan. 1948): 32–33, 82, 84; Geister, "Candid Comments on the Spirit of Nursing," *RN* 12 (Nov. 1948): 31–33, 72, 74, 76, 78; Geister, "Candid Comments: America Loves Numbers," *RN* 16 (Sept. 1953): 38–39; Geister, "Weighing the Quality of Nursing," *RN* 16 (Dec. 1953): 49–52, 61; Geister, "Patients, Procedures, and Projects," *RN* 18 (June 1955): 43, 46, 72; Alice R. Clarke, "Transition vs. Tradition," *RN* 19 (Nov. 1956): 44–45.

56. Ada L. Burt, "Antibiotics Improve Nurse-Patient Relationships—No," *Nursing World* 125 (July 1951): 290; letter from Dolores T. Keydrash, Halethorpe, Md., *RN* 16 (Dec. 1953): 14.

57. Letter from Mary Parker Lowry, Yuba City, Calif., *RN* 10 (Aug. 1947): 7; Janet M. Geister, "Man's Inhumanity to Man," *RN* 12 (Dec. 1948): 30–32, 68, 70; letter from R.N., Washington, D.C., *RN* 12 (March 1949): 10; Pearl E. Wilson, "Why Don't They Listen?" *RN* 16 (Oct. 1953): 38–39, 82; letter from Jeannette Newhall, Fulton, Mo., *RN* 11 (Nov. 1947): 6, 8, 10.

58. Arthur J. Geiger, "In Unions There Is Strength?" *RN* 3 (Dec. 1939): 10–13, 28–29.

59. Letter from R.N., Oakland, Calif., *RN* 6 (Nov. 1942): 2; letter from Mary Shea, Seattle, Wash., *RN* 4 (July 1941): 2; letter from Charlotte S. Dubois, Mt. Rainier, Md., *RN* 10 (Oct. 1946): 8, 10; see also letter from R.N., Elyria, Ohio, *RN* 10 (Nov. 1946): 7; letter from Caroline E. Renneker, *RN* 10 (Dec. 1946): 7; letter from Dorothy L. Trice, Brooklyn, N.Y., *RN* 10 (Dec. 1946), 8, 10; letter from Mary E. Jones, Goodnight, Okla., *RN* 10 (March, 1947): 7. For a provocative interpretation of labor in the 1950s, see George Lipsitz, *Class and Culture in Cold War America: "A Rainbow at Midnight"* (New York: J. F. Bergin Publishers, 1982).

60. Letter from R.N., Dayton, Ohio, *RN* 9 (Dec. 1945), 10, 12, 14; letter from R.N., Chicago, Ill., *RN* 4 (July 1941): 2; letter from R.N., Detroit, Mich., *RN* 5 (Dec. 1941): 4; letter from R.N., New York, *RN* 6 (Feb. 1943): 2. See also letters from Detroit, *RN* 4 (May 1941): 2–3; Berkeley, Calif., *RN* 5 (June 1942): 6, 8; Philadelphia, *RN* 6 (Oct. 1942): 6, 8; Springfield, Ill., *RN* 6 (May 1943): 6; Cecelia Konefal, Buffalo, N.Y., *RN* 6 (May 1943): 6, 8.

61. "Economic Security Program: Balloting," *Pacific Coast Journal of Nursing* 39 (April 1943): 115–18; and see monthly progress reports in the same journal, June through October, which culminate in the announcement of successful mediation in favor of CSNA.

62. Daniel H. Kruger, "Bargaining and the Nursing Profession," *Monthly Labor Review* 84 (July 1961): 699–705.

63. Letter from R.N., Chicago, *RN* 4 (July 1941): 2; letter from R.N., Detroit, *RN* 4 (Sept. 1941): 6, 8; letter from R.N., Pontiac, Mich., *RN* 9 (June 1946): 7.

64. Quotation from Emma Harling, "The Vanishing Heart of Nursing," *RN* 19 (Oct. 1956): 53–54, 84. For examples of the growing emphasis on the nurse-patient relationship (and the new enthusiasm for the social sciences), see Hildegard E. Peplau, *Interpersonal Relations in Nursing* (New York: G. P. Putnam's Sons, 1952); Frances Cooke MacGregor, *Social Science in Nursing* (New York: Russell Sage, 1960).

65. Editorial, "Changes in Nursing Practice," *AJN* 47 (Oct. 1947): 655 (encourages staff nurses to submit nursing care studies to the journal); Margaret Strom Schubert, "Case Discussions with Student Nurses," *AJN* 48 (Jan. 1948): 29–32; Marie E. Nielsen, "Case Method of Assignment," *AJN* 49 (Sept. 1949): 576–79; Dorothy M. Smith, "Patient-centered Teaching in Medical and Surgical Nursing," *AJN* 50 (May 1950): 314–15.

66. June S. Rothberg, "Why Nursing Diagnosis?" *AJN* 67 (May 1967): 1040–42; Basil S. Georgopoulous and Luther Christman, "The Clinical Nurse Specialist: A Role Model," *AJN* 70 (May 1970): 1030–39; Marie Manthey et al., "Primary Nursing: A Return to the Concept of 'My Patient, My Nurse,'" *Nursing Forum* 9, no. 1 (1970): 64–83; A. M. Robinson, "Primary Nurse: Specialist in Total Care," *RN* 37 (April 1974): 31–35; Karen L. Ciske, "Accountability—the Essence of Primary Nursing," *AJN* 79 (May 1979): 890–94; Mary O'Neil Mundinger, *Autonomy in Nursing* (Germantown, Md.: Aspen, 1980); Karen S. Zander, *Primary Nursing* (Germantown, Md.: Aspen, 1980).

67. Marlene Kramer, *Reality Shock: Why Nurses Leave Nursing* (St. Louis: Mosby, 1974).

CONCLUSION

1. For information about the numbers and proportions of nurses with degrees, see Nursing Information Bureau, *Facts about Nursing*, (New York: American Nurses' Association, 1965), p. 63; N.I.B., *Facts about Nursing* (New York: ANA, 1970), p. 77; "New Records," *RN* 35 (April 1972): 5, 7; "Who Works Where at What?" *RN* 37(June 1974): 42. For contemporary discussion and debate about the increasing emphasis on degrees, see Stella Goostray, *Memoirs of Half a Century of Nursing* (Boston: Boston Univ. Nursing Archives, 1969), p. 152; "1965 NLN [National League for Nursing] Convention," *American Journal of Nursing* (hereafter cited as *AJN*) 65 (July 1965), 108–13; Verle Hambleton Waters, "Distinctions Are Necessary," *AJN* 65 (Feb. 1965), 101–2; Wanyce C. Sandve, "Diploma Programs Need Scrutiny," *AJN* 65 (Feb. 1965): 103–4; Patsy Lane Williams Winter, "I Am Not a Technician," *AJN* 65 (May 1965): 130. See also letters columns

filled with the debate in *AJN* for Feb., April, May, July, and Aug. 1965. For a report on and criticism of the New York State Nurses' Association's action for a more restrictive credential, see Glen Jenkins, "1985: Closing the Door on Nurses, New York Style," Health Policy Advisory Center *Bulletin* 78 (Sept./Oct. 1977): 1–7.

2. Letter from Patricia A. Stephens, R.N., Denver, Colo., *RN* 32 (Sept. 1969): 18; letter from Dorothy Nafis, R.N., Savannah, Ga., *RN* 33 (Feb. 1970): 22. For letters from nurses critical of baccalaureate nurses, see Frances Chlystun, R.N., Lexington, Ky., *RN* 30 (Sept. 1967): 19; Barbara J. Dillon, R.N., Virginia Beach, Va., *RN* 32 (March 1969), 11; Madrea J. Hudson, R.N., M.S., Tallahassee, Fla., *RN* 39 (Sept. 1976): 135–36.

3. "ANA Asks Equal Pay for AD and Diploma Nurses," *RN* 30 (Feb. 1967): 25; "Diploma RNs Rated Tops by Nurse-Employers," *RN* 39 (Oct. 1976): 8; "ADs May Apply!" *RN* 34 (July 1971): 9; "Barriers Down!" *RN* 35 (Aug. 1972): 5.

4. For a discussion of recent innovations in the organization of health care, see Elliott A. Krause, *Power and Illness: The Political Sociology of Health and Medical Care* (New York: Elsevier, 1977), especially part two, "Patterns: The Systems of Care and Neglect," pp. 123–220. For early examples of independent nursing practice, see "Nurse Teams Hang Out Their Shingles," *AJN* 74 (Jan. 1974): 10; Betty C. Agree, "Beginning an Independent Nursing Practice," *AJN* 74 (April 1974): 636–42; Judith D. Jordan, "A Nurse-Practitioner in Group Practice," *AJN* 74 (Aug. 1974): 1447–49. And for a recent account, see Karon White Gibson, Joy Smith Catterson, and Patricia Stalka, *On Our Own* (New York: St. Martin's Press, 1981).

5. "Taft-Hartley Changes Due," *AJN* 74 (Sept. 1974): 1209–10; "Taft-Hartley Amendments Become Law; Hospital Exemption Ended," *AJN* 74 (Sept. 1974): 1560–61.

6. Lauren Crawford and Pat Circzyc, "Nightingales Strike," *Health-Right* 3 (winter 1976–77): 1, 6; "Providence Nurses Win Voice in Policy Making," *AJN* 76 (Feb. 1976): 181; Joan Yeager, "Why I Had to Strike," *AJN* 77 (May 1977): 874. See also "ANA Pleased with Strike Settlement," *AJN* 74 (Aug, 1974): 1387, a report of a California strike: "The fundamental issue of the strike, as the ANA understands it, was the issue of patient care—whether or not nurses themselves determine the quality of nursing care which the patient receives." A recent manual of workplace organizing is written by and directed to nurses: see Karen O'Rourke and Salley Barton, *Nurse Power: Unions and the Law* (Bowie, Md.: Robert J. Brady Co., 1981).

7. For a discussion of recent organization of hospital workers, including nurses, see Richard U. Miller, *The Impact of Collective Bargaining on Hospitals* (New York: Praeger, 1979).

8. Letter from Nurses Now, *AJN* 74 (March 1974): 423.

9. Classic theoretical statements of this viewpoint are cited in Introduction, note 6; major historical interpretations that take this perspective are

Louise A. Tilly and Joan W. Scott, *Women, Work, and Family* (New York: Holt, Rinehart, and Winston, 1978), and Leslie Woodcock Tentler, *Wage-Earning Women: Industrial Work and Family Life in the United States, 1900–1930* (New York: Oxford Univ. Press, 1979).

10. For recent studies that emphasize the strength of women's work culture and female commitment to work, see Susan Porter Benson, " 'The Clerking Sisterhood': Rationalization and the Work Culture of Saleswomen in American Department Stores, 1890–1960," *Radical America* 12 (March–April 1978): 41–55; Thomas Dublin, *Women at Work: The Transformation of Work and Community in Lowell, Massachusetts, 1826–1860* (New York: Columbia Univ. Press, 1979); and Evelyn Nakano Glenn, "The Dialectics of Wage Work: Japanese-American Women and Domestic Service, 1905–1940," *Feminist Studies* 6 (fall 1980): 432–71.

Index